A Woman's Guide to Total Wellness

A Woman's Guide to Total Wellness

The Balanced Approach to Live Well, Age Beautifully

Mia Cowan
MD, FACOG, MA, MBA

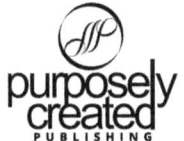

A WOMAN'S GUIDE TO TOTAL WELLNESS
Published by Purposely Created Publishing Group™
Copyright © 2017 Mia Cowan

All rights reserved.

No part of this book may be reproduced, distributed or transmitted in any form by any means, graphics, electronics, or mechanical, including photocopy, recording, taping, or by any information storage or retrieval system, without permission in writing from the publisher, except in the case of reprints in the context of reviews, quotes, or references.

Most of the information in this book is taken from years of reading, learning, practicing gynecology, weight loss, and hormone replacement therapy, and training at the Center of Medical Weight Loss and Biote.

Printed in the United States of America
ISBN: 978-1-948400-34-3

Special discounts are available on bulk quantity purchases by book clubs, associations and special interest groups. For details email: sales@publishyourgift.com or call (888) 949-6228.

For information logon to:
www.PublishYourGift.com

Dedication

A Woman's Guide to Total Wellness is dedicated to you, my Ageless Belles!

Table of Contents

Introduction 1

SECTION 1:
MAINTAINING A HEALTHY WEIGHT 3

Secret #1: Protein is Power 5

Secret #2: Counting Calories Counts 13

Secret #3: The Scale NEVER Lies 17

Secret #4: Don't Skip Breakfast 21

Secret #5: Eat Several Small Meals + Snacks 25

Secret #6: Don't Waste Water! 29

Secret #7: Exercise Is Necessary for Weight Maintenance and Enhances Weight Loss 35

SECTION 2:
DEVELOPING A HEALTHY LIFESTYLE 41

Secret #8: Clean Eating Decreases Your Exposure to Toxins 43

Secret #9: Adequate Sleep Is Necessary for Total Wellness 47

Secret #10: Stress 51

Secret #11: Supplements Help Prevent Disease 55

Secret #12: Meal Replacements Aid in Nutrition and Calorie Control 59

Secret #13: Make Good Choices in Tough Situations 63

Secret #14: Plan, Shop, and Prep to Maintain a Healthy Lifestyle 67

SECTION 3:
BALANCING FEMALE HORMONES 71

Secret #15: Menopause 73

Secret #16: Testosterone 77

Secret #17: Estrogen 81

Secret #18: Thyroid 85

Secret #19: Weight Gain 89

Secret #20: Mood 93

Secret #21: Sex Drive 97

SECTION 4:
VISITING YOUR GYNECOLOGIST/PREVENTION .. 101

Secret #22: Pap Smear Recommendations and
               Annual Exams 103

Secret #23: Fibroids/Bleeding 107

Secret #24: Finished Having Babies, Now What? 111

Secret #25: Adolescents and the Gynecologist 113

Secret #26: Vaginal Maintenance 115

Secret #27: Breast Cancer 117

Secret #28: Heart Disease 119

About the Author 123

Introduction

Welcome Ageless Belles.

My name is Dr. Mia, and I am a board-certified gynecologist and your B3 specialist. I have created MiaCowanMD.com to help women who are struggling with weight gain, fatigue, and low sex drive improve their **B3: beauty, balance, and belief** through education and cutting-edge medicine.

This book gives you my TOP secrets to take a beautiful approach to health through balance and belief, to live well, and to age beautifully. Belles, after reading this book, you will live your best healthy life. You will learn my secrets to maintaining a healthy weight, developing a healthy lifestyle, increasing your inner energy, and balancing your female hormones. You will learn tips that most gynecologists won't even tell you. These secrets have worked for me, so as a doctor, I KNOW they will work for you too. I practice what I teach. Let's learn, ladies.

Dr. Mia

SECTION 1

Maintaining A Healthy Weight

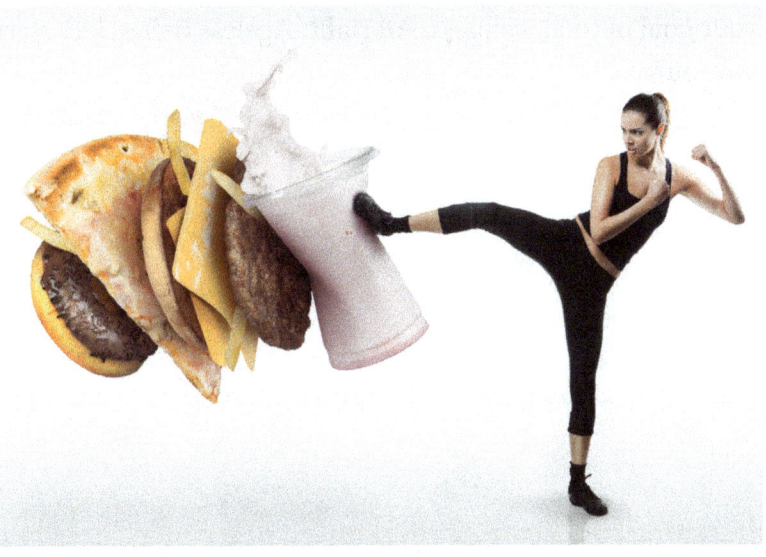

This section will teach you to attain and maintain a healthy weight. As we all know, we have all lost weight on several different occasions, and we know it can become more difficult with age, but imagine losing weight the right way, through modifying behavior, monitoring calories, and living a healthy lifestyle to keep it off forever. It becomes very stressful to your body to continually lose and gain weight, which has a negative impact on your health, metabolism, and weight. Remember—it's important to make behavior modifications to improve metabolism, but maintaining weight loss requires good mental health, healthy coping skills, exercise, a healthy and balanced diet, meditation, emotional and spiritual intelligence, and hormonal balance. In this section, you will receive my best tried-and-tested advice to accomplish your goal of total wellness. All right, Ageless Belles, let's start our journey!

SECRET #1

Protein Is Power

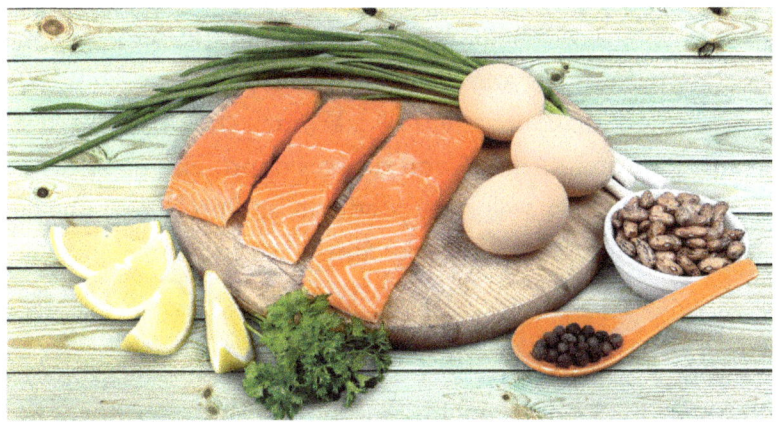

Maintaining a healthy weight can be very difficult and becomes harder as we age. As we age, we naturally lose about a pound of muscle each year after the age of 25, which negatively affects our metabolism—hence the reason we tend to gain weight in our mid-20s. As our muscle mass declines, so does our metabolism, making it easier for us to gain weight. To better control metabolism, it is necessary to eat frequent small meals, avoid skipping meals, eat adequate protein, and drink plenty of water. Many of my patients notice a 5 to 15 pound weight gain between ages 20 and 25. Other times when women gain significant weight are during your late 30s and early 40s, the freshmen 15, and let's not forget, menopause. Basically, we are always working to maintain a healthy weight, so here is some information that will make this journey easier.

Adequate protein in your diet keeps you satiated or full longer and helps control cravings so you consume fewer calories. Protein also helps you maintain muscle, which is important to improve your metabolism, so you lose weight faster and maintain your weight loss. Women should eat 60 to 80 grams of protein a day. Good sources of protein include lean meat, eggs, beans, soy, dairy products, and protein on the go, such as meal replacement protein shakes and bars.

Meat

I recommend eating organic meats to ensure that there are no added hormones or harmful preservatives, which are more expensive but still healthier. As you can see with the list of protein options below, it's easy to get plenty of protein with lean meat. Try steaming, grilling, baking, or sautéing your meat in a nonstick pan.

- **Chicken** – Chicken breasts are the best option from chicken because they contain less fat than the thigh, leg, and wing. If you choose to eat chicken, remove the skin and as much of the visible fat as possible when preparing the meat for seasoning to help decrease your fat and calorie intake. Preparing the chicken on the grill, in the oven, and even on the stovetop with only a small amount of olive oil with the pan top in place will keep the chicken juicy and more flavorful. When seasoning chicken, use fresh herbs and vegetables to cut down on the need for salt for flavor. For each ounce of chicken breast, there are about 7 to 8 grams of protein, so one 3.5-ounce chicken breast has 140 calories and 30 grams of protein, compared to a chicken thigh, which has 217 calories and only 16 grams of protein.

- **Seafood** – Seafood has variable amounts of protein: salmon has 149 calories and 21 grams of protein as compared to red snapper, which has 145 calories and 29 grams of protein; 4 ounces of shrimp has 67 calories and 28 grams of protein; 4 ounces of catfish has 108 calories and 20 grams of protein; and 4 ounces of raw cod has 120 calories and 26 grams of protein.

- **Red meat** – Red meat has more saturated fat and should be eaten infrequently. Limiting red meat decreases your risk for heart disease and colon cancer. Try to avoid rib eye, porterhouse, and T-bone steak to improve your protein-to-fat ratio. Healthier options include eye of round, the sirloin tip side, top sirloin, bottom round, and skirt steak. I'm not saying you can't enjoy a steak every so often, but I would limit that consumption to two to four times per month and choose the healthier options with plenty of protein and less fat. For example, a 4 ounce piece of filet mignon has 216 calories, 4 grams of saturated fat, and 32 grams of protein, compared to a 4 ounce top sirloin with 210 calories, 5 grams of saturated fat, and 23 grams of protein. A 4-ounce rib eye steak has 330 calories, 11 grams of saturated fat, and 27 grams of protein.

- **Pork** – Two pieces of pork bacon have 80 calories, 3 grams of saturated fat, and 5 grams of protein compared to two pieces of turkey bacon, which have 60 calories, 1 gram of saturated fat, and 4 grams of protein. Limit your pork consumption to decrease calories and saturated fat. Turkey is a good substitute.

Dairy

Milk, cheese, and yogurt are also good sources of protein, however, it is necessary to monitor the fat and sugar when looking at the nutrition facts. Greek yogurt, with 140 calories or lower with 10 to 15 grams of protein per serving, has more protein than plain yogurt and is a great meal replacement. I am lactose intolerant, so I use almond milk or coconut milk and ice cream. I limit my cheese consumption, but I find that I have fewer symptoms with feta cheese compared to some of the other options.

Other

There are several other protein options that can be used in smoothies and recipes:

- **Soy** – Soy is used as a protein substitute; 4 ounces of tofu has 86 calories, 1 gram of saturated fat, and 9 grams of protein.

- **Eggs** – Eggs are a great source of protein and nutrition. They can be boiled, scrambled, over easy or made into an omelet with veggies. Eating the whole egg provides the most protein; the egg whites only have 3 grams of protein, compared to 7 grams in the whole egg. Don't forget about egg salad and adding eggs to recipes for protein and flavor.

- **Beans** – One cup of black beans has 227 calories, no saturated fat, and 15 grams of protein; red beans have 206 calories, no saturated fat, and 12 grams of protein.

- **Protein Additives** – Additives are great for smoothies. Whey protein is a mixture of globular proteins extracted from whey, which is created as a by-product of cheese production, hence the reason some people experience bloating. Pea protein is made from peas and works well for people with lactose intolerance. I prefer to use a gluten-free protein powder to decrease bloating and gas.

As you can see, there are many ways to get lean protein in your diet to help maintain your muscle and improve your metabolism to make it easier to maintain your healthy weight. Remember, eat everything in moderation. I find that when I say I can't have it, I crave it more. When choosing protein-rich foods, look for low-calorie foods with adequate protein and minimal saturated fat and sugar. Reading labels is key to monitoring your nutrition intake and, most importantly, measuring and weighing your portions make it much easier to stay within your calorie range so you can maintain total wellness.

> **HOMEWORK:** Go grocery shopping at your local organic store and purchase chicken breasts, etc. Try steaming, grilling, baking, or sautéing your meat in a non-stick pan. Use fresh herbs and vegetables for flavor. Yummy! I find that I stick to my calories and protein better when I eat a variety of foods with new and different recipes. Try some of the recipes below and add your own twist, focusing on nutrition, calories, and portion control.

1. Smoothie recipe with kale, protein powder, and fruit:

    2 scoops of protein powder

    1 cup of almond milk

    ½ cup of frozen strawberries

    ½ banana

    ½ cup of kale and blueberry mix

    Blend to desired consistency.

    Calories: 230

    Protein: 20 grams

2. Chicken teriyaki over brown rice and veggies:

   Chicken breast, seasoned with salt and pepper

   Frozen veggies with broccoli, cauliflower, and carrots; Grilled fresh veggies (onions, red, yellow, and green peppers, sautéed in 1 tablespoon of olive oil, cooked covered on medium for 5 minutes)

   Brown rice cooked as directed

   Teriyaki sauce (low sodium)

   Brown meat after seasoning, and add sautéed veggies; once cooked, add frozen veggies; steam on medium to cook veggies after adding teriyaki sauce to desired taste. One cup of stir fry and ½ cup of brown rice is 550 calories and 30 grams of protein.

3. Grilled shrimp with sweet and sour sauce over veggies: Sauté onions, red and green peppers in olive oil and add 1 pound of deveined and shelled shrimp. Cook on medium-low with pan top in place for 5 to 7 minutes. Add sweet and sour sauce over frozen veggies in a different pan and cook for 7 to 10 minutes once tender. Add veggies and sauce to cooked shrimp with sautéed veggies. Two cups contain 450 calories and 25 grams of protein.

4. Filet mignon meal: 4-ounce steak with 1 cup of sweet potato and salad with 2 tablespoons of vinaigrette dressing. Grill steak to preferred temperature. Bake sweet po-

tato until tender throughout. Add 1 tablespoon of butter and side salad with vinaigrette dressing. Contains 550 calories and 25 grams protein.

5. Blackened red snapper with asparagus:

    Cajun seasoning mix: 1 teaspoon each of paprika, onion powder, cayenne pepper, ground black pepper, dried thyme, dried oregano, and 1 tablespoon of kosher salt

    2 tablespoons of olive oil

    2 tablespoons of butter

    1 lemon

    Mix Cajun seasoning and sprinkle over cleaned and dried fish. Add fish to hot skillet with butter and olive oil. Cook on each side until blackened and done in center for 5 minutes each side. Grill asparagus with salt and pepper. Six ounces of red snapper and two cups of asparagus contains 350 calories and 41 grams protein.

SECRET #2

Counting Calories Counts

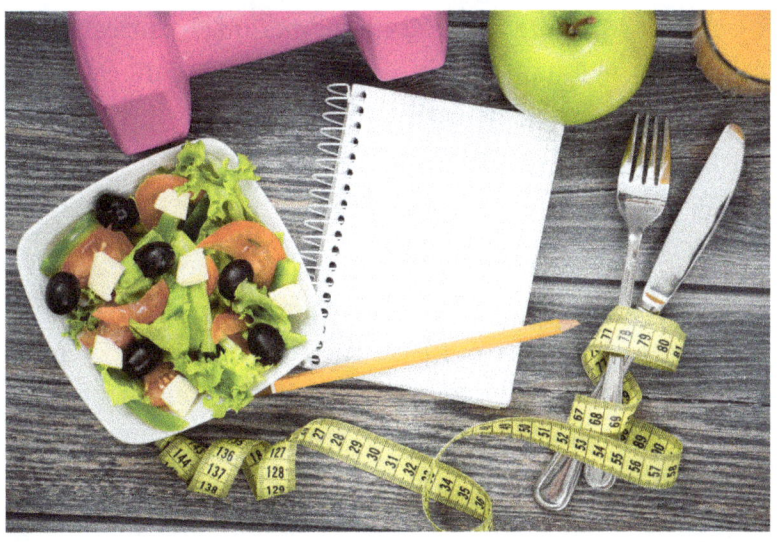

I know. You hate counting calories! But if you know your metabolic rate and stay within your calorie range, it helps you lose weight faster and maintain the weight loss. It's not as hard as it sounds. If you use an app on your phone, monitor, and journal your calories obsessively for one month, it will become second nature. Remember to measure and weigh your food for more accuracy. Once you reach your weight loss goals, continue to monitor your calories to maintain your new healthy weight.

I recommend you do a resting metabolic rate test to determine how many calories you need to eat to lose weight and maintain weight. For example, I completed the test, and I know that my resting metabolic rate is 1440, which means I burn 1,440 calories in a 24-hour period. I can eat 1,440 calories to maintain weight, however, I can only eat 1,100 to 1,200 calories when trying to lose weight. This takes all the guessing out of my weight management, allowing me to reach and maintain my weight goals.

I also had a genetic test done, which shows that I lose weight faster by doing a balanced diet and minimizing my fat. Through trial and error, I have learned what foods keep me satisfied longer and the foods that make me hungry throughout the day. This information is important because I know to hold off on sugars and carbs until later in the day so that I don't snack all day and go over my calories. This is why journaling is so important in the beginning of your weight loss journey, because you can review your journal to see what has worked best for you over the month as far as calories and foods that keep you satisfied longer and allow you to stay in your calorie range.

There is a huge difference in empty calories and nutritious calories. Empty calories have no real nutritional value, meaning no fiber, protein, or healthy fat; and nutritional calories do have fiber, protein, and healthy fat. For example, when you eat a 100-calorie snack pack of pretzels (empty calories) compared to an apple and ½ tablespoon of peanut butter (nutritional calories), you are eating the same number of calories, however, you will be satisfied for two to three hours after the apple compared to 30 to 60 minutes with pretzels. Pretzels are empty calories with no real nutritional value, but the apple has fiber and vitamins, and the peanut butter has healthy monosaturated fats. Examples of healthy, nutritional snacks are almonds, Greek or regular yogurt, veggies and hummus, grapes and nuts, a variety of different fruits, turkey-wrapped string cheese, a small bowl of fiber cereal and milk, and a nut mix.

> **HOMEWORK:** Journal your food for one week and see how many calories and grams of protein you eat. Weigh yourself at the beginning of the week and weigh yourself again after a week of journaling. Add to your journal how you feel at the end of the day, e.g., any unexpected hunger surges and any increased energy. Note how satisfied you are after each meal and document when you feel hungry so you can see which foods keep you satiated longer. Use one of the free food journaling apps on your smart phone.

SECRET #3

The Scale NEVER Lies

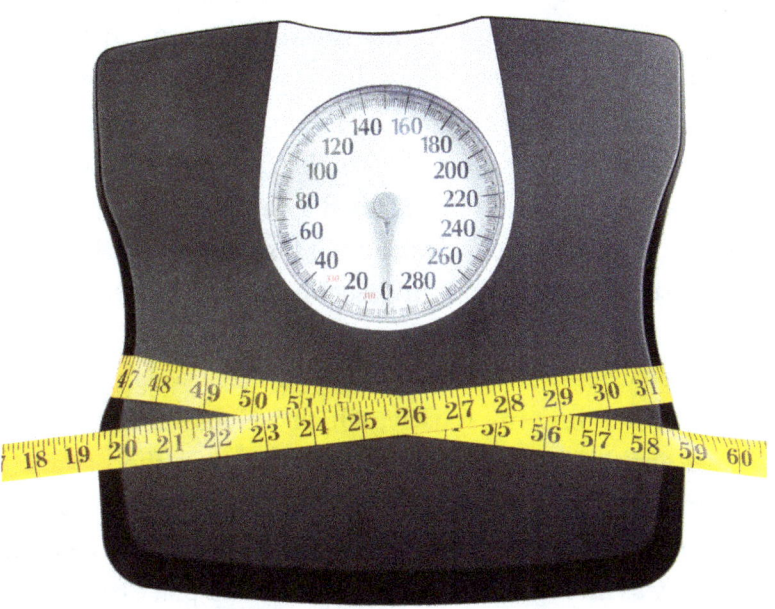

Knowing your weight is essential to maintaining a healthy weight because numbers don't lie! I know a lot of Belles hate getting on the scale, but weighing yourself at least once a week helps you monitor changes. It is much easier to lose 2 to 3 pounds compared to 10 to 15 pounds! Remember, our clothes stretch, but numbers don't tell untruths! Weigh yourself first thing in the morning. Do this before eating or drinking and after eliminating overnight wastes (urinate and have a bowel movement before weighing, if possible). I personally weigh daily because it keeps me focused on making healthy choices.

In the past, it has been difficult for me to lose weight. I tried it every way I could, but I failed miserably not counting my calories and going over my calorie recommendations. I began reaching my weight goal because I started to measure, weigh, and journal. I measure and weigh my food for portion control and I journal my calories throughout the day. Most importantly, I plan my meals for the day so I can stay in my calorie range, and I can continue to lose the weight to reach my personal goal of not only reaching a healthy weight but also looking and feeling good. I notice that when I work out more consistently, I don't see a huge drop in weight because I am maintaining my muscle, which weighs more than fat. To stay encouraged, monitor your weight on the scale but also monitor your measurements. Measure your waist at the belly button, your mid-thigh and mid-upper arms, as well as hips. Try to measure your inches in the same place each time. For example, measure 5 inches above your knee each time, 4 inches above your elbow, and around the largest circumference of your hips.

It is important to know your body mass index, which is easily calculated on several apps or through a formula. Once you calculate your BMI, try to stay in the normal weight range to decrease your risk of heart disease, cancer, and diabetes! If your BMI is 18.5 to 24.9, you are considered normal weight. If your BMI is 25 to 29.9, you are considered overweight. If your BMI is 30 to 39.9, you are considered obese, and a BMI of 40 or higher is morbid obesity.

Have a scale to weigh yourself regularly and have your body composition analyzed regularly to ensure that you are losing fat and not muscle. I have a body composition analysis scale at my office that shows muscle mass, water percentage, weight, BMI, and basal metabolic rate. There are similar scales that are more affordable and can help you monitor your overall progress. Many times when doing weight training and having adequate testosterone, the muscle mass improves, which weighs more than fat and the drop in pounds are not as obvious, but a body composition scale allows you to see if there is an improvement in muscle, which is key to long-term weight loss. At the very least, have a scale that you weigh on regularly, at least once a week, so you can monitor any change in your weight. You can also monitor your measurements with a measuring tape or with the fit of a pair of jeans. People who weigh regularly maintain their weight better than people who rarely weigh.

> **HOMEWORK:** Calculate your BMI and determine how many pounds you should lose to get in the normal weight range. Determine the frequency of weighing yourself that fits with your lifestyle and personality. I recommend once a week, but that causes anxiety for some people, so at the very least, weigh twice a month.

SECRET #4

Don't Skip Breakfast

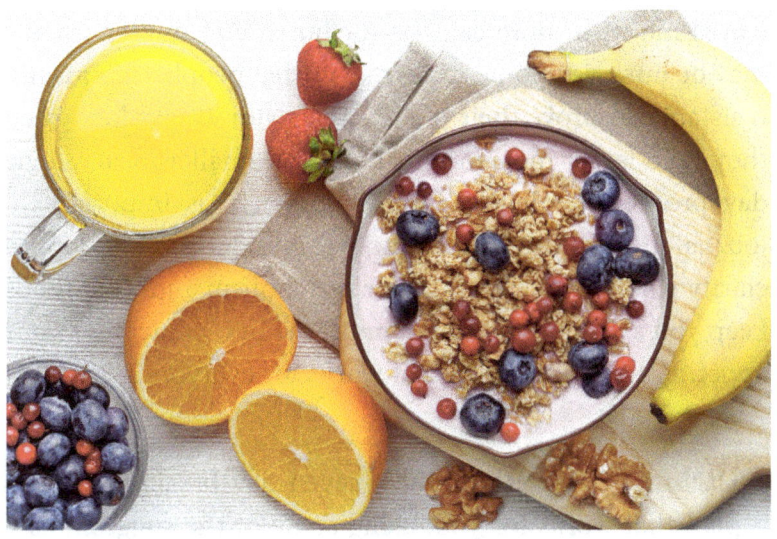

Breakfast is the most important meal of the day, and to be considered breakfast, it should be eaten within the first hour of waking up! Your breakfast should include plenty of protein and healthy fat to start your metabolism for the day, which makes it easier to lose weight. Skipping breakfast puts your body in starvation mode, and for the rest of the day, your body will store all calories as fat to ensure enough energy for the day, causing you to gain weight. My patients with the most challenging weight issues skip breakfast on a regular basis. Make breakfast a priority and follow it with frequent small meals throughout the day.

If it's difficult for you to eat earlier in the day, eat a light breakfast and save those calories for other meals. For example, some mornings I have one or two boiled eggs, but that leaves me with more calories for lunch and dinner when I may be hungrier. Some studies show that people with insulin resistance improve their blood sugars and weight loss when they eat a larger meal for breakfast and smaller meals as the day progresses. Hence, another reason it is important to journal food, calories, and hunger surges. Journaling helps to clarify what works best for your metabolism and what foods keep you satisfied so you can make the best choices for your appetite. There is no plan that works for everyone.

> **HOMEWORK:** Write out a seven-day breakfast meal plan that works for you, using some of the suggestions below. Go grocery shopping for the week after you write out your meal plan. Make sure you measure, weigh, and journal serving size, calories, and protein to make it effortless during the busy week. Remember to plan ahead so you stick to the plan.

1. 2 boiled eggs
2. Greek yogurt and high protein granola and/or fruit
3. Protein smoothie
4. 2 egg omelet
5. Eggs and bacon
6. Ready made protein shake or bar
7. Steel cut oatmeal with fruit

SECRET #5

Eat Several Small Meals + Snacks

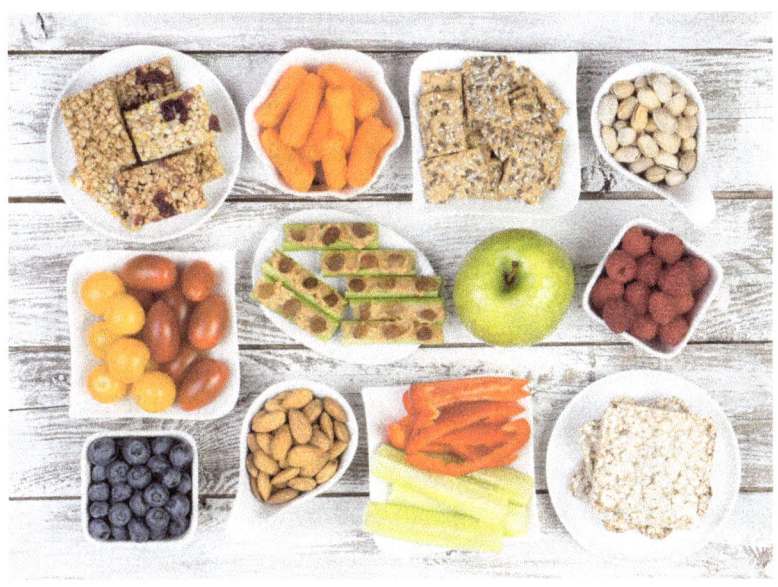

The higher your metabolism, the easier it is to lose weight and then maintain a healthy weight. You should eat five to six small meals a day. Eat breakfast within the first hour of waking up; then eat a small meal every two to three hours. When you eat frequently, your body uses those calories for energy right away instead of storing them as fat, keeping your metabolism revved up to help you maintain a healthy weight.

When I monitor my calories, I usually have a protein shake in the morning (180 to 275 calories, 20 grams of protein), and for my morning snack, I have eight to ten almonds with water or a piece of fruit; for lunch I may have a smoothie with 450 calories, or a salad with 450 calories, all with 15 to 25 grams of protein. I would then eat fruit or nuts for my snack, staying in the range of 50 to 150 calories and for dinner, a smoothie or meal replacement like Greek yogurt, grilled chicken and veggies, or a small portion of a meal, limiting portion size to 300 calories or less with 20 grams of protein. Some people hate meal replacement shakes and bars and prefer to eat actual meals, which works well as long as you plan ahead and monitor your calories, protein, and serving size. Studies have shown that people who eat one to two meal replacements a day tend to maintain their weight loss better.

As you can see, I stay satisfied by eating lean, high-protein foods frequently, with plenty of hydration to decrease hunger surges and improve metabolism.

> **HOMEWORK:** Go shopping for fruits, veggies, and snacks. Add a meal plan for lunch for seven days. Here are some examples below. Use simple recipes with lean meat, protein, and healthy fat. Use one of your apps to determine calories, protein, and serving sizes as you make your favorite recipes.

1. Tuna salad lettuce wraps with fruit on the side: Minimize the mayo and substitute with Greek yogurt to decrease fat and add protein. Use fresh tuna or albacore tuna in the pack with water instead of the canned tuna.

2. Grilled chicken and salad: Put dressing on the side. Use a vinaigrette dressing and measure the serving size. Add plenty of raw, fresh veggies to the salad for more fiber and satiety.

3. Protein shake: Use almond milk and a protein substitute or Greek yogurt. I prefer a little sweetener for added flavor; agave nectar works well and has a low glycemic index.

4. Turkey chili; Use your preferred chili recipe with chili powder, black beans, pinto beans, tomato paste, and chili flavored tomatoes. Don't forget about fresh veggies, like onions and bell peppers, to improve the flavor of the ground turkey.

5. Turkey spaghetti: Use your preferred recipe substituting ground beef with ground turkey. Make sure you drain the cooked meat. Instead of spaghetti sauce, use tomato paste, fresh and canned tomatoes, and wheat noodles.

6. Chef salad with egg, chickpeas, and beans, and/or lean turkey meat: Choose a low-calorie dressing and measure out the serving size. Keep dressing on the side so you use less.

7. Chicken salad on a green salad with limited pita chips: Use chicken breast, and substitute some of the mayo with Greek yogurt. Use fresh onions and pickled relish for flavor and measure your recipe for calorie and protein accuracy.

SECRET #6

Don't Waste Water!

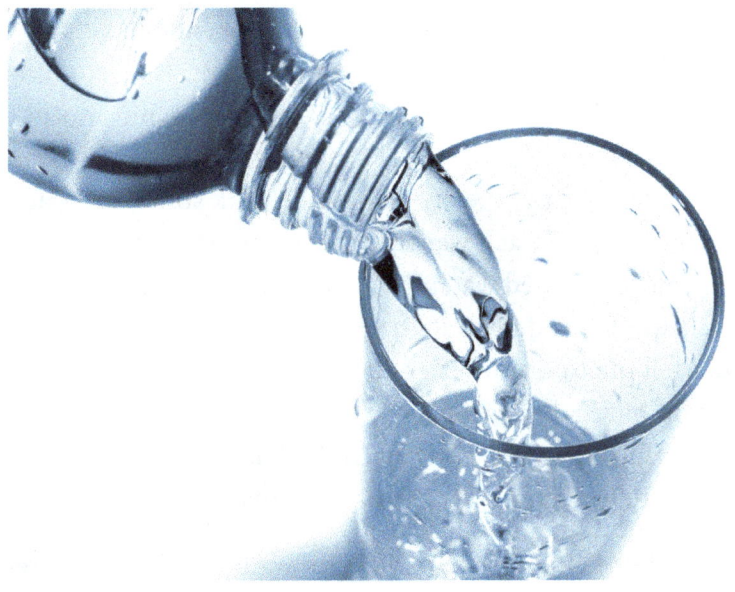

You should drink at least half your weight in ounces of water every day, up to 100 ounces. Water keeps you hydrated and decreases hunger. I recommend drinking 16 to 20 ounces of water with each meal. Drink half of it before you start eating and complete the other half before you finish your meal. Being thirsty can mimic hunger, so always drink a few ounces of water if you feel hungry before it's time for your next meal. If you had a meal an hour and a half ago and you are feeling hungry sooner than you expected, try drinking 16 to 20 ounces of water and wait 10 minutes before eating a snack early; many times, you will forget that you were "hungry."

By staying hydrated with water and minimizing sugar and salt in your diet, you tend to have fewer hunger surges. Many times our bodies tell us we are hungry, and in actuality we are thirsty and need some good ole water. It's a running family joke that water cures all, according to my mother. My mother is a nurse of over 40 years, and whenever I complained of anything, she always said, "Drink some water and rest!" So if my stomach was upset, I was constipated, or I was dehydrated, I needed water; if I had a headache, I needed water because I was dehydrated, and if I was oversnacking, she would tell me to drink water. And she was on to something! So if you have a headache, feel fatigued, have problems with constipation or an upset stomach, try increasing your water intake to relieve many of those symptoms.

Another benefit is that adequate water intake helps tremendously with weight loss and maintenance. I hear a lot of my weight loss patients say they don't like water (which is quite baffling to me because it has no taste), so I recommend drinking it at room temperature to drink it faster and just get the proper amount down. I also recommend drinking it cold with clean fruit or veggies for flavor, such as lemons, cucumbers, strawberries, kiwi, orange slices, or lime slices, or other pieces of fresh fruit.

Avoid Crystal Light and other flavor packets with sugar or sodium because they can still make you hungrier and more dehydrated. Although artificial sweeteners don't have calories, they can still have a high glycemic index, which makes you hungrier. Seltzer water expands your stomach and makes you hungrier. The cups that maintain temperature are great to carry around so you always have cold water with you especially in the summer. I make sure I have water with me at all times, and I keep it well stocked at home and at the office. It is initially frustrating to have to frequent the bathroom, but the more consistent you are with getting your water in daily, your bladder adjusts, and though you still go often, it does improve with time.

Here is a breakdown of the different types of water:

- **Tap water** that is unpurified has more than 300 different pollutants and should be avoided.

- **Spring water** quality varies greatly and contains naturally occurring minerals and trace elements like magnesium, sodium, zinc, calcium, potassium, and selenium, to name a few, but in very small quantities.

- **Bottled water** can have purified and unpurified tap water. If it is purified, it will say it on the label, but it is really just expensive tap water. Sometimes you may only have the option of purified bottled water, however, filtered tap water is just as good and less expensive.

- **Distilled water** does not have the healthy minerals or impurities in tap water because they have all been removed. It tends to have a bland taste but can be used occasionally to cleanse the body.

- **Carbon filtration** is a good way to get healthy water for much cheaper. Carbon filters remove many of the harmful chemicals from tap water.

- **Ozonated water** is sterilized drinking water. Ozone destroys bacteria, fungi, algae, and viruses. Home ozonater systems remove odors and chemicals.

- **Plain drinking water** is much better than any of the waters with flavor or electrolytes; and as I said earlier, plain water with a slice of fruit or a vegetable will quench your thirst and help the taste if you have a hard time just drinking plain water.

- Gatorade and Power-aide, as well as artificially sweetened beverages and flavor packs, should be avoided.

Remember to drink water before each meal and complete your water prior to finishing your meal and you may eat a lot less.

> **HOMEWORK:** Cut out sodas, juice, and other sugary beverages. Drink half your weight (pounds) in ounces of water, up to 100 ounces/day. For example, if you weigh 160 pounds, drink 80 ounces of water per day.

SECRET #7

Exercise Is Necessary for Weight Maintenance and Enhances Weight Loss

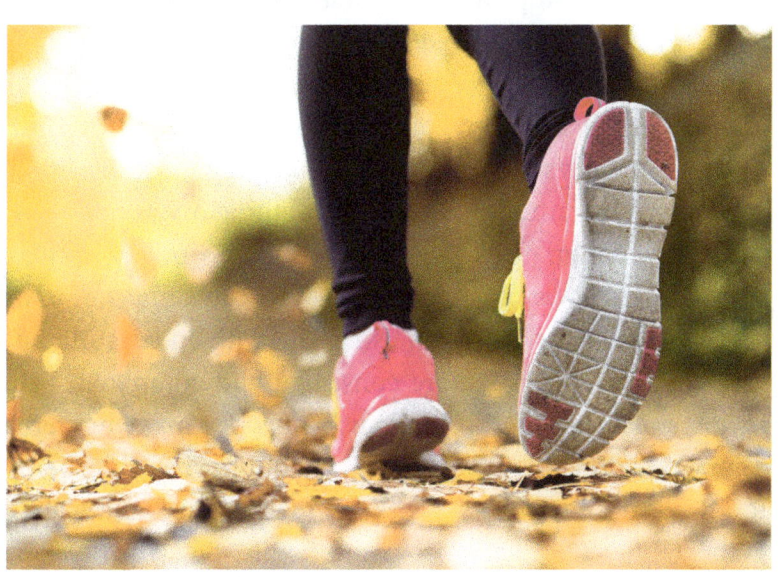

Exercise plays a huge role in the maintenance of healthy weight. Though it is important to include cardio, it is even more important to incorporate resistance training, like Pilates, weight training, calisthenics, swimming, and yoga into your exercise regimen for muscle and bone maintenance. Remember, we naturally lose muscle as we age, however, incorporating resistance training into your training helps you maintain muscle. This is important because maintaining muscle improves metabolism, making it easier to lose the weight and keep it off.

We all know that exercise alone won't control your weight, but the combination of consistent exercise and healthy eating will improve your health and weight management. Exercise is also good for improving mood, sleep, and energy. For me to get my exercise in consistently, I have learned through trial and error that I have to schedule my workout for the early morning in my home and pay a trainer to make sure I get up three to four days per week for a challenging workout. If you can't afford a trainer, I recommend finding a workout buddy, joining a gym near your home, going to workout classes, or purchasing workout videos that you can do at home or when traveling. I find that working out with an accountability partner makes me more consistent and compliant. I do my personal training with my husband while my daughter is asleep! My previous excuses included not having time, being too tired to exercise after work, hating the gym, and feeling guilty taking time away from my family. So with my new routine, I have no excuses! Exercising 150 to 180 minutes a week is a reasonable goal. However, as I age, I find that I need to work out almost daily for an hour and include resistance training as well as cardiovascular training. We all have barriers to exercise, so it is necessary to find ways to work around those barriers because exercise is necessary for total wellness and graceful aging!

Exercise is so important for several reasons:

- It improves muscle tone, balance, and stability.
- It improves mood and energy by releasing natural endorphins.
- It improves flexibility, bone mass, weight loss, and maintenance.
- Cardio training helps strengthen the heart, improve stamina, and burn calories.
- Resistance training helps significantly with muscle mass, metabolism, bone mass, balance, flexibility, and strength.
- The combination of cardio training with resistance training helps significantly with overall weight management, health, and total well-being.

> **HOMEWORK:** Design a workout plan you can do at home or in a hotel room and use some of the suggestions below. Most importantly, try sticking to the plan for 21 days.

Start with 15 to 25 reps of at least four different exercises that you can do daily and continue to add five reps each week or every other week:

- **Push-ups** can be done the traditional way, with your knees on the floor (aka girl push-ups), or standing with arms on the wall. As the arms get stronger, you can improve to the more advanced push-ups. Start with 10 and continue to increase each week. I had to initially break up my push-ups into sets until my arms got stronger.

- **Sit-ups** the old-fashion way are better for working more of your abdomen. Start with 10 and work your way up to 25. Feel free to do sets of 10 to 15.

- **Jumping jacks** can be done the traditional way if you don't have knee problems. Or, they can be done without jumping by stepping out to the right with the right foot and raising the right hand (like the arm motion with regular jumping jacks) then doing the same on the left. Try doing them as quickly as possible to increase your heart rate.

- **Squats** can be done with a chair, but be sure to not allow your knees to go over your toes. Stand in front of the chair, squat down to let your bottom touch the chair, and then immediately stand up with your feet shoulder length apart.

- **Lunges** can be done walking and alternating feet, or they can be done one leg at a time, ensuring that your knees don't go over your toes. .

- **Mountain climbers** work well to increase your heart rate and work your entire body. With hands on the floor and feet on the floor, alternate moving your feet on your tiptoes, keeping your hands in place on the floor.

- **Burpies** are difficult, so start with as little as five and move up. Start by lying on your stomach and using your arms to push up and stand. If advanced, you can jump as you stand to your feet. Burpies work the entire body and give you cardio and resistance training all in one. Increase by two to five each week.

SECTION 2

Developing A Healthy Lifestyle

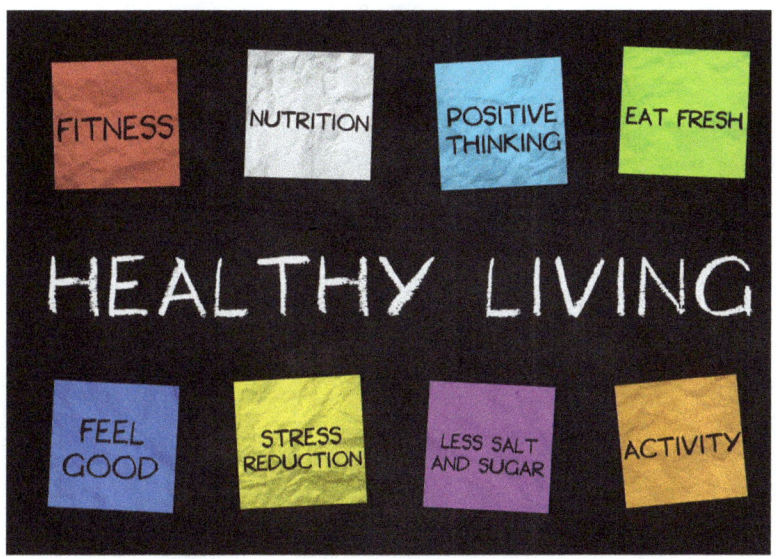

Total wellness not only requires developing a healthy weight and maintaining it. Total wellness also requires developing a healthy lifestyle, including choosing healthy, clean foods, getting adequate rest, being emotionally healthy, practicing mindfulness, taking proper supplements, and living an overall healthy lifestyle to ensure that you are able to enjoy your beauty, balance, and belief so you can live well and age beautifully. All right, Ageless Belles, let's continue on our journey to total wellness!

SECRET #8

Clean Eating Decreases Your Exposure to Toxins

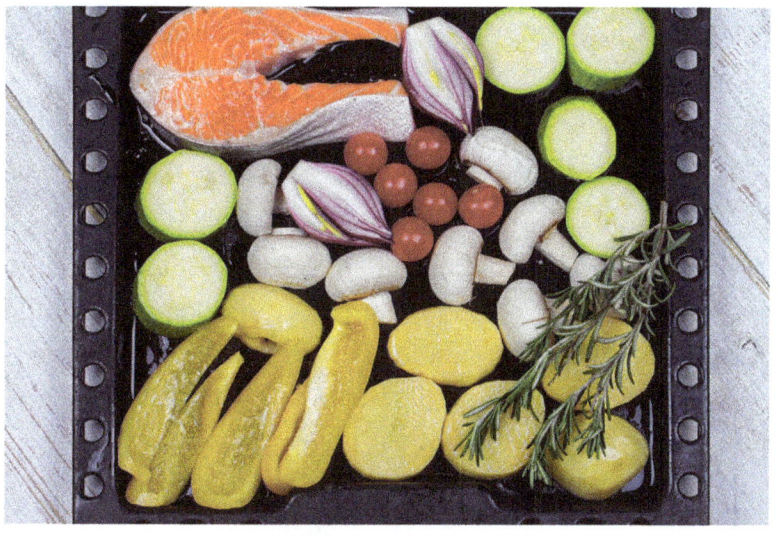

Choosing healthy foods and a diet rich in protein and fiber will help you maintain a healthy weight and keep you from overeating. Avoid white rice, bread, pasta, and potatoes, as well as processed foods, as much as possible. Substitute the white stuff, or simple carbohydrates, with brown rice, sweet potatoes, wheat bread, and wheat pasta, which contain more complex carbohydrates. Also, increase your intake of fruits, nuts, and vegetables. Eat more vegetables that are dark green such as broccoli, spinach, and leafy greens. Include orange vegetables like carrots and sweet potatoes, as well as dry beans like peas, black beans, pinto beans, and lentils. Try to eat lean meat free of hormones and avoid processed foods with added preservatives, sugar, and salt. In other words, try to eat the foods Adam and Eve likely ate when first put on Earth, such as lean protein, fruits, vegetables, nuts, and seeds. But just because we choose to eat clean and healthy does not mean that we can eat as much of it as we want. We must still monitor calories and portion sizes to stay within our calorie range to lose those extra pounds.

Conventionally raised poultry has been shown to contain several additives including caffeine, Prozac, and arsenic, to name a few. By choosing certified organic foods, it should minimize exposure to antibiotics, hormones, and heavy metals. There are several labels associated with alternatives to conventionally raised poultry:

- **USDA Organic Certification**: Inspected by a USDA-accredited inspector who has ensured that the farm followed federal requirements that chickens were raised without antibiotics, were fed 100 percent organic, and had "reasonable access" to outdoors.

- **Free-Range Certification**: Chickens with this label had access to the outdoors for more than half their lives.

- **Pastured**: Means chickens are housed at night and are free to roam during the day, but there is no legal definition.

> **HOMEWORK:** Go grocery shopping and pay attention to nutrition labels. Try to purchase clean foods and foods with natural fiber.

SECRET #9

Adequate Sleep Is Necessary for Total Wellness

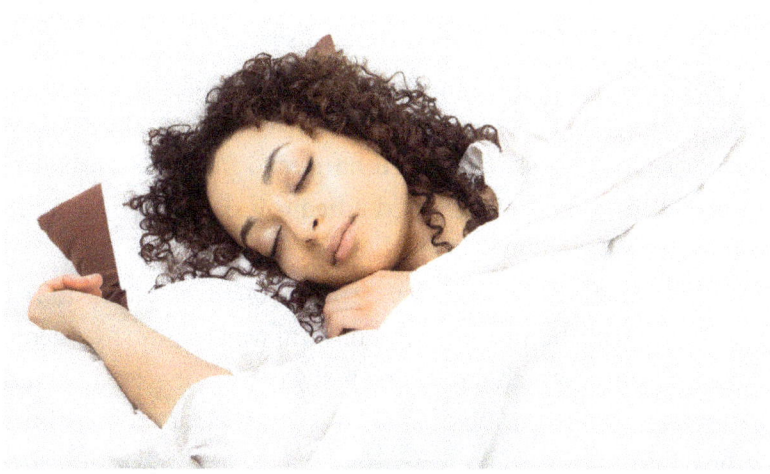

You should be getting seven to nine hours of sleep per night. If you are having problems sleeping, have a sleep study to ensure that you don't have sleep apnea. Avoid caffeine late in the evening and maintain a healthy sleep environment, void from noise and electronics. Also, have your testosterone levels checked because low testosterone and hormonal imbalance can cause insomnia. Many of my patients start having problems with sleep in their mid to late 30s, which is about the time that testosterone starts to decline for many women. Low testosterone affects sleep and energy, as well as sex drive and orgasms. Replacing testosterone has allowed many of my patients to have complete resolution of insomnia and now they are more rested and can avoid addictive prescription sleep medications. Restful sleep improves overall quality of life and health, as well as mood, weight, and energy.

As you may know, when you don't get enough sleep daily, you put out extra cortisol because your body becomes stressed with lack of rest, and you start gaining weight in your mid-section. These elevated cortisol levels make it much harder to lose weight and even harder to maintain a healthy weight. Once you have created a healthy sleep environment, made behavior changes and balanced your hormones, you should notice a huge improvement in your rest. Melatonin 1 mg three hours before sleep is a natural way to improve sleep. Avoid alcohol, which can worsen sleep, and obviously avoid caffeine later in the day. Also, limit liquids closer to bedtime. If possible, turn off all electronics that could make noise or flashing lights, which can easily interrupt your sleep. Close all doors in your bedroom and turn off all lights. Also, wear your CPAP if diagnosed with sleep apnea and comply with all recommended treatment.

Did you know that heart disease is the number one cause of death? Did you also know that sleep apnea is one of the top causes of heart disease? Sleep apnea decreases oxygen to your heart, which can eventually lead to irreversible lung and heart disease and, eventually, death. Obesity increases the risk of heart disease, obstructive sleep apnea, and death. Maintaining a healthy weight improves your sleep, and restful sleep makes it easier to maintain a healthy weight.

> **HOMEWORK:** Practice getting seven to nine hours of sleep a night. Have a sleep study, clean up your sleep environment, and try to go to sleep at the same time every night if possible to establish a good sleep routine.

SECRET #10

Stress

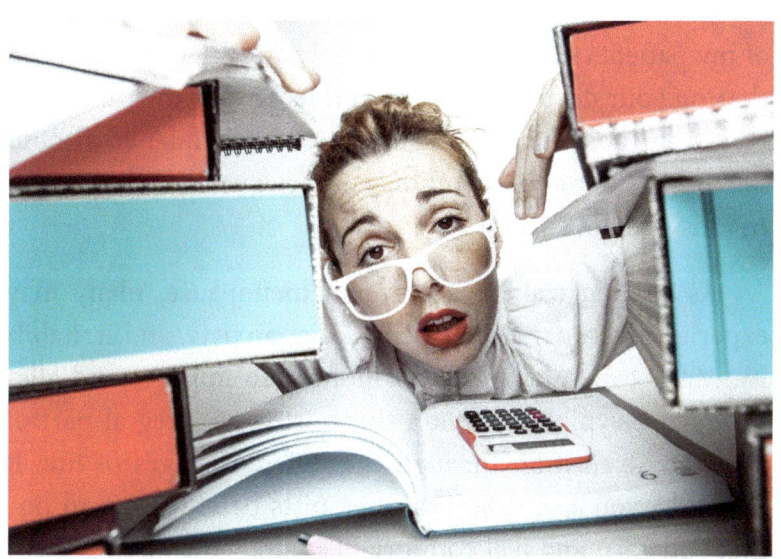

Stress management is key to health. Examples of ways to manage stress are:

- Exercising regularly
- Seeing a therapist regularly
- Meditation and yoga

Many of my patients downplay the importance of a therapist, and I always remind them that they have to take care of their minds as much as their bodies. As we age, we all experience significant stress, and coping skills are not innate; most people need help and training to cope with stress. A trained professional who is unbiased, can't share your deepest thoughts with anyone else, and can help you see other perspectives is an integral part of a healthy lifestyle. Some of my patients say they talk to family and friends, but when sharing your deepest thoughts and feelings with a therapist, you know those feelings will be shared in confidence without the judgment and bias you may experience from family and friends who love you.

As women transition through menopause, many may experience an increase in depression, anxiety, and irritability. Many times, balanced hormones can improve and alleviate these symptoms, but a therapist is an integral part of a healthy transition through the different stages of life. It may take you seeing several therapists before you find one that you trust and feel comfortable with, which is why I encourage my patients to seek out a good therapist as soon as possible and well before they actually need one. Insurance sometimes covers therapy, but there are many programs that may assist with the cost of therapy. In fact, some churches and nonprofit groups offer therapy at a discounted rate or sometimes at no charge.

- **Massage** is a wonderful way to relax and relieve stress. I recommend a massage one to four times per month. It's a great way to be in a quiet place and clear your mind. This can be done at a cheaper rate at massage therapy schools and massage centers.

- **Meditation** generally takes training but is a great way to clear your mind. Even five minutes a day of meditation can improve health and relieve anxiety. There are several mobile apps that can help train you to meditate.

- **Mindfulness** is also a great way to relieve stress and anxiety. Mindfulness allows you to focus on the moment and not the past or future. In other words, you must slow down and stay present, which can increase happiness and decrease stress. There are many books that teach mindfulness.

- **Yoga** is a good way to train yourself to meditate and be mindful, and it is a great way to exercise and improve your balance and flexibility. Furthermore, finding a hobby you enjoy, like running, playing an instrument, fishing, or golfing, will help alleviate stress and improve your quality of life and happiness.

- **Intentional Relaxation** requires you to use a day or two every quarter to simply relax and only do the things you truly enjoy *without electronics or a cell phone*. Allow yourself to enjoy a restful day each quarter to feel renewed.

> **HOMEWORK:** Start meditating and practicing mindfulness. Start with five minutes, three times a week until it becomes a part of your everyday life.

SECRET #11

Supplements Help Prevent Disease

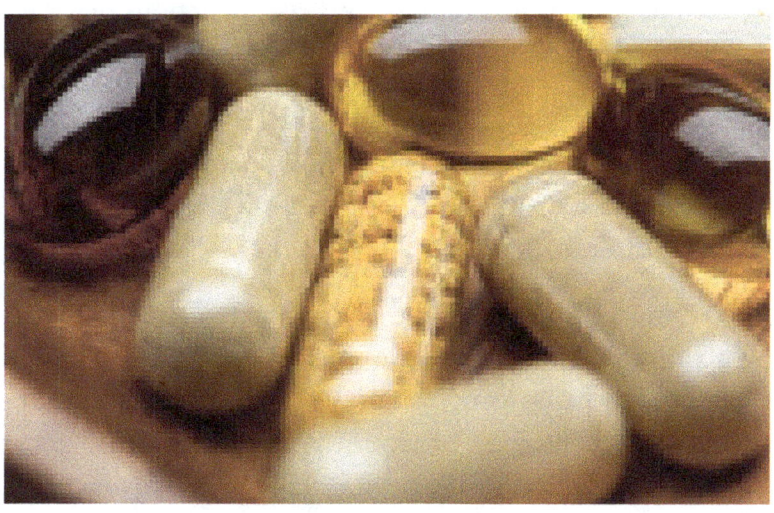

I recommend my Belles over the age of 40 to take omega-3 daily because it improves heart health and cholesterol, decreases joint pain, and improves depression, ADD, and other neurological disorders. Make sure that you choose an omega-3 with adequate long-chain fatty acids, EPA (eicosapentaenoic acid) and DHA (docosahexaenoic acid), for better absorption. There is a prescription omega-3, with DHA and EPA, that works really well. Ask your doctor about it. Also, omega-3 is naturally found in cold-water fish, shell fish, plant nuts, oils, flaxseed, English walnut, algae, and fortified foods.

Probiotics are live bacteria and yeast that occur naturally in your gut to help to increase bowel movements for detoxification and help your immune system fight disease. Probiotics help alleviate symptoms associated with irritable bowel syndrome, inflammatory bowel disease, infectious diarrhea, and diarrhea from antibiotics.

CoQ-10 improves energy, mental clarity, and heart health. I recommend my patients on statin drugs for high cholesterol take CoQ-10, as well as, if they have high blood pressure or heart disease.

Vitamin D3 levels should be maintained at 60 to 70 ng/ml to improve energy, decrease bone loss, improve mood and sleep, and decrease your risk of cancer and multiple sclerosis (MS). I recommend replacement with Vitamin D3 either daily or weekly depending on your level. Over 40 percent of Americans have low levels of Vitamin D, so I recommend regular screenings of Vitamin D levels to ensure adequate replacement. I also recommend a Vitamin D3 with Vitamins A and K for better absorption. Calcium intake has been shown to aid in both weight loss and bone health.

> **HOMEWORK:** Start with two different supplements listed above that would help your total health. Continue to add until you are taking all supplements that will improve your total health and wellness.

SECRET #12

Meal Replacements Aid in Nutrition and Calorie Control

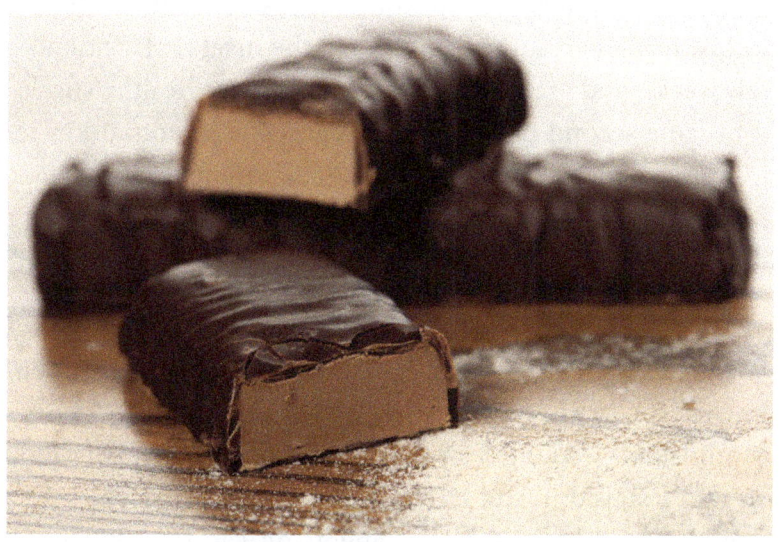

Meal replacements are key to weight loss and maintenance. A good meal replacement has 150 to 250 calories and 10

to 30 grams of protein. The purpose of meal replacements when initially starting a healthy diet to lose weight, is to shrink your stomach, so you can't overeat. When I initially lost my weight, I had a meal replacement shake or bar for breakfast and lunch, a light morning and afternoon snack, and a healthy meal with my family for dinner. Sometimes, I would eat a meal for lunch and have a protein shake for dinner, which worked well also. After doing this for two to three weeks, I was at the point where it was difficult to overeat, and if I did, it made me sick.

The biggest hurdle with weight loss is changing behaviors so that it becomes natural to incorporate the new behavior into your daily routine. After doing the meal replacements a few weeks, and eating a healthy meal and two healthy snacks, it became second nature. Also, meal replacements aid in retraining your taste buds to enjoy foods without a lot of sugar, fat, and salt.

My metabolism increased with the frequent, small meals, and I was never hungry because I ate plenty of lean protein and fiber, which kept me satisfied. I also began to enjoy healthy food again, and my fast food and sweet cravings diminished. I counted my calories and journaled my food so that I stayed in my 1,100 calorie range for weight loss. I would even take meal replacements on vacation, but I still enjoyed a meal or two out each day while minimizing eating too many calories. When on vacation, the goal is to not gain weight. Don't stress yourself out with trying to lose weight on vacation; just maintaining your weight is a reasonable goal. Examples of meal replacements include two boiled eggs, turkey and cheese, Greek yogurt, and protein bars and shakes.

> **HOMEWORK:** Try several different meal replacements that have at least 20 grams of protein and under 200 calories. Be creative and choose foods that can serve as a meal replacement but aren't typical meal replacement bars and shakes. For example: Greek yogurt, fresh fruit, and protein granola.

SECRET #13

Make Good Choices in Tough Situations

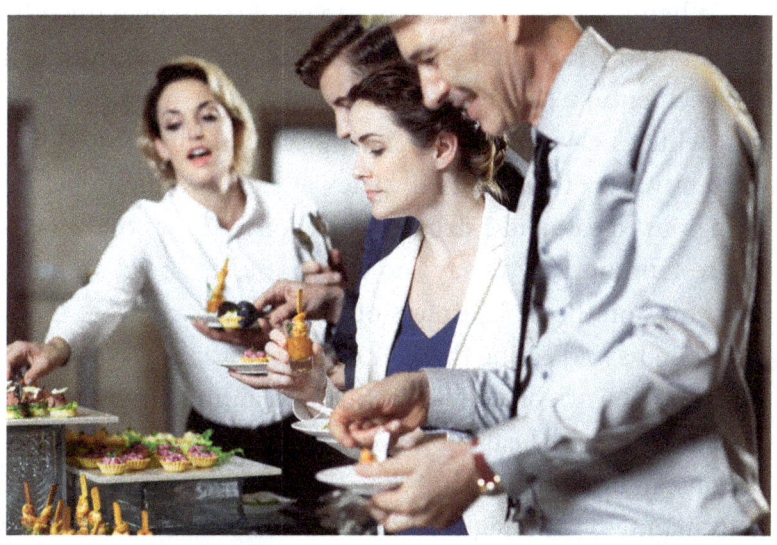

Of course, I have tried almost every fad diet out there, but I learned a few years ago that if I wanted to lose weight and keep it off, I had to make some lifestyle changes. I began to pay attention to nutrition facts, try new recipes and meal replacements, and switch up my meal choices to see what worked best for me. I always look at the calories and protein, and monitor the amount of sugar and salt in my meals. I try to avoid eating out frequently so that I don't have to make hard choices, however, it is inevitable that I eat out at restaurants because of my lifestyle. Before I go to a restaurant, I preview the menu and try to choose a restaurant with healthy options. I remember to avoid bread, simple carbs, cream sauces, and dessert (most times).

When I know I am going out to eat, I try to plan my other meals so I eat small frequent meals, incorporating meal replacements so that I save up calories for the meal I will eat out, which helps me to stay in my calorie range. Most importantly, I try to eat a small snack at least two hours before going out to eat, and I drink a bottle of water on the way to the restaurant. I try to say "no thank you" to bread and tortilla chips on the table, unless others in my party want them and then I avoid eating them or only have a small taste. I also make sure I work out extra when I am planning to eat out at a restaurant in case I eat a few more calories than planned. Vacation can be a challenging time to stay on plan. So my goal is to maintain my weight and increase my exercise by either going to a gym at the hotel, exercising in my room, or staying active in the pool or with walking tours.

When I drink alcohol, I try to avoid sweet drinks like margaritas and piña coladas and opt instead for either a light beer, liquor on the rocks, or a low calorie beverage, if I decide to have a drink. I have also learned to attend social events with the intention to socialize and not eat. If I do eat, I taste fresh fruits and veggies and minimize the higher calorie appetizers and desserts. I drink a bottle of water or glass of water for every alcoholic beverage I drink to stay hydrated and drink and eat fewer calories.

> **HOMEWORK:** Go out to a restaurant to eat, preview the menu, and choose a dinner under 500 calories that you enjoy. Plan before you go and stick to the plan. It is inevitable to eat out occasionally, so practice making good choices in difficult situations.

SECRET #14

Plan, Shop, and Prep to Maintain a Healthy Lifestyle

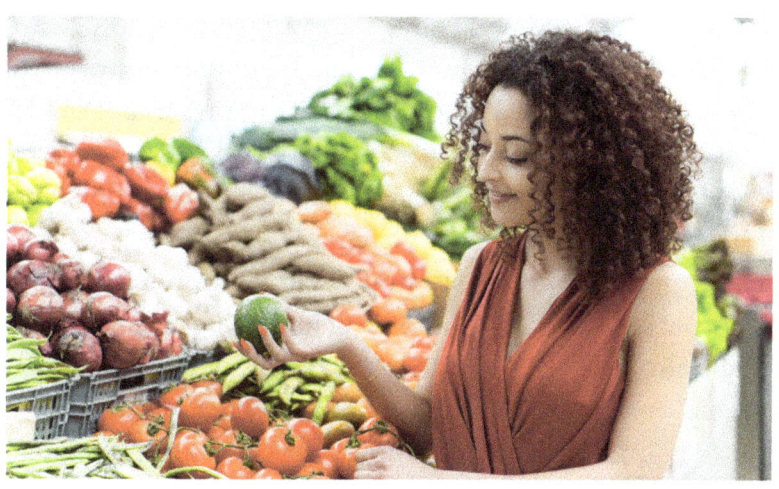

Planning and prepping meals are keys to a healthy lifestyle. We try to do our grocery shopping on the weekend and plan our meals for the week. When purchasing meat, it is easier to immediately weigh it and separate it in a freezer bag, labeled with weight and calories, so when preparing meals through the week, it is easier to count calories. We did a poor job of planning initially, but now we order from one of the companies that deliver all the ingredients to our doorstep, and we cook at least three home-prepared meals per week, which allows us to eat most meals at home when including leftovers. We chose a company with organic meats, high-quality vegetables, well-balanced meals, and a good variety of healthy meals. And of course, you can plan your meals for the week and do your grocery shopping on the weekend yourself, as well as prepare some of your meals on the weekend. Once my meals are planned for the week, I make sure I have access to healthy snacks and water so that I eat small meals every two to three hours throughout the week. I find that keeping fruit around helps my sweet tooth, and it's always a low-calorie snack that I can eat quickly to ensure that I never go over three hours without eating. I also keep almonds around, and I like apples and bananas with almond butter every so often. Healthy snacks with fiber, healthy fat, and protein tend to keep me satisfied longer. Instead of just eating an apple I may add 8 almonds or ½-1 table spoon of peanut butter. I dip my veggies in hummus and I keep protein bars on hand, even if I only eat a ½ for my morning snack and finish the other half for my evening snack. As long as I have access to healthy snacks and meals, I easily continue my healthy lifestyle. However, I have caught myself slipping, and ended up without available snacks, which is when I am more likely to make unhealthy choices, causing me to go over my calories for the day. When I plan and prepare appropriately, some days I bring a light lunch, such as a protein shake, which gives me time to incorporate a walk during lunch. When I exercise at lunch, I have more energy in the afternoon, and I eat fewer calories, so I can enjoy a better dinner with my family.

> **HOMEWORK:** Plan your meals, snacks, and exercise for the week. Stay within your recommended calorie and protein goals and try to get in some exercise during lunch. Take light meals or meal replacements. Purchase snacks, meals, and ingredients for the week and stick to the plan.

SECTION 3

Balancing Female Hormones

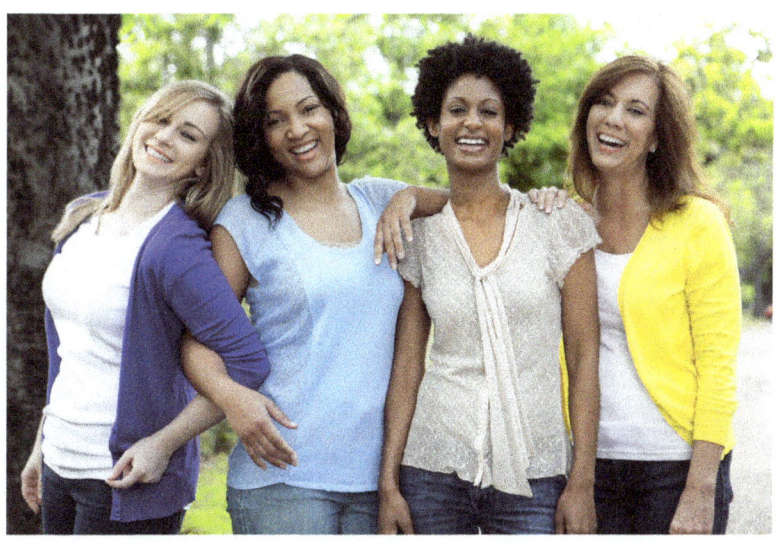

Our hormones play a huge role in our health, as well as our quality of life. As we age our hormones change and decline, which can cause symptoms of fatigue, weight gain, decreased sex drive, decreased orgasm, vaginal dryness, irritability, depression, anxiety, hot flashes, night sweats, and problems with sleep. These changes can be caused by imbalanced testosterone, progesterone, estrogen, thyroid, neurotransmitters, and vitamins. It is necessary to monitor these symptoms because if they are consistent, your hormones may be out of wack, which can also increase your risk of heart disease, bone loss, dementia, and other chronic illnesses. Hormonal balance improves your health and quality of life so you can live well and age beautifully.

SECRET #15

Menopause

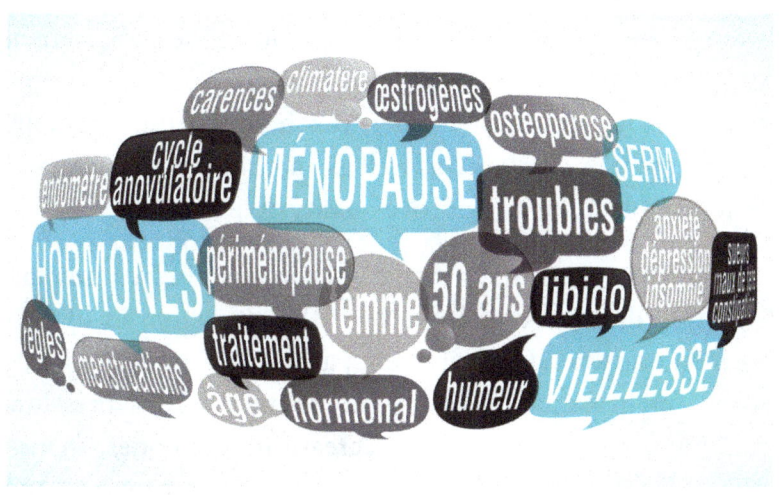

A woman is considered postmenopausal when she stops having cycles for a year, her ovaries are surgically removed, or her ovaries stop functioning, per a blood test. Women can have symptoms of menopause up to 10 years prior to menopause. Menopausal symptoms include hot flashes, night sweats, mood changes, anxiety, depression, fatigue, decreased sex drive, difficulty sleeping, weight gain, and vaginal dryness. These symptoms can be attributed to low estrogen, progesterone, and testosterone. Adequate hormone replacement can alleviate these symptoms and improve your overall health.

Menopause can be a very difficult transition for women, and it is the beginning of the aging process. Lack of hormones increases the aging process, whereas replacement of hormones usually slows the aging process. As you know, all women are not good candidates for hormone replacement therapy, which includes estrogen, progesterone, and testosterone. However, most women can benefit from hormone replacement and balance as well as vitamin replacement and other supplements to improve quality of life.

I recommend that women prepare themselves mentally, physically, and emotionally for this transition in life. As women transition through menopause, many notice a significant weight gain, worsening fatigue, increased depression, and anxiety. Because of the decrease in hormones, menopausal women have an increased risk of heart disease and bone loss. I encourage my patients to develop a healthy lifestyle well before transitioning into menopause to maintain total wellness and to age gracefully. I recommend for women having gynecological surgery to maintain their ovaries, provided they are normal, because in doing so, they do not incur significant health risks.

Many women in America have hysterectomies, however, it is important to explore all options. Fortunately, with technological advances, there are several minimally invasive procedures that don't require the removal of the uterus and will still alleviate abnormal bleeding. After a hysterectomy, some women tend to experience menopausal symptoms earlier, even when the ovaries are not removed. I recommend my patients keep their ovaries if they don't have a strong family history of breast or ovarian cancer, as long as they are normal. Removing ovaries early increases the risk of mortality and morbidity from heart disease and bone loss. A lot of women think that it is easier to have everything removed during a hysterectomy to avoid future surgery, when in actuality, less than 10 percent of women who keep their ovaries ever need reoperation. There are special cases like a family history of breast, ovarian, or uterine cancer tied to a genetic mutation that significantly increase the risk of cancer. Many women get their ovaries removed, not understanding the possible negative effects on their quality of life. Many women with surgical menopause experience more severe symptoms like hot flashes, night sweats, vaginal dryness, mood changes, decreased libido, mood changes, fatigue, and insomnia. Women under the age of 60 with a low risk for cancer based on personal history and family history should keep their ovaries as long as they are normal. This allows a more natural transition into menopause, and decreased mortality and morbidity associated with heart disease. Transitioning naturally through menopause can be very difficult, but a natural transition may be more tolerable for many women.

HOMEWORK: Journal your symptoms for one to two weeks. Journal how much you are sleeping and resting, how many calories and grams of protein you're intaking, how many ounces of water you are drinking, and any symptoms (along with the frequency and severity) discussed above, such as fatigue, mood changes, night sweats, mind fog, weight gain, hot flashes, insomnia, or joint pain. If you notice that your symptoms are affecting your quality of life, see a gynecologist who specializes in hormone balance and total wellness.

SECRET #16

Testosterone

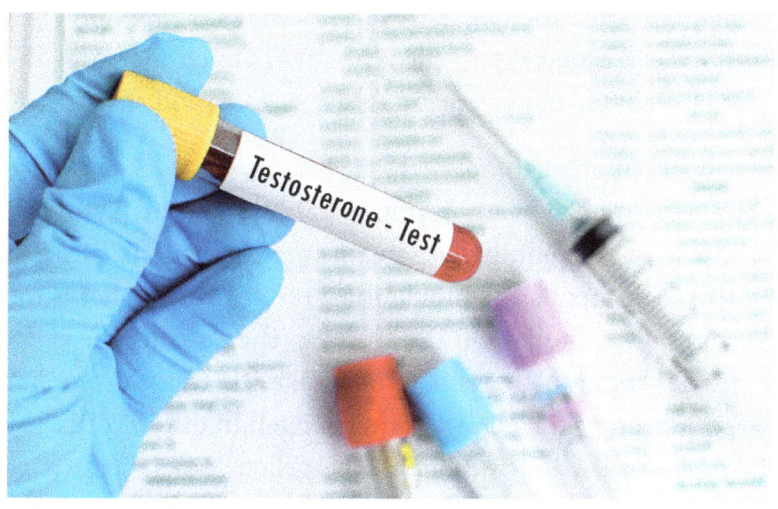

Testosterone is the forgotten female hormone, and when it is low, women may experience mood changes, decreased sex drive, night sweats, decreased orgasm, fatigue, weight gain, joint pain, decreased focus and memory, and problems sleeping. Women under 40, as well as postmenopausal women, can experience these symptoms secondary to low levels of testosterone. Replacing testosterone not only alleviates these symptoms, but adequate testosterone levels decrease the risk of heart disease, bone loss, and dementia. Many women begin to experience these symptoms in their late 30s and find themselves on medications like antidepressants, anxiety medications, diet pills, medications to improve focus, blood pressure medications, sleep medications and diabetic medications. However, many times the real issue is lack of testosterone, which effects mood, memory, weight, energy, sleep and sexual function. As testosterone decreases, weight tends to increase, especially in the abdomen, which increases the risk of diabetes, hypertension, heart disease, and stroke.

Testosterone can be safely replaced either with a testosterone cream or pellet for women, although other synthetic forms exist, including gels, creams, and injections, which I don't recommend. The bioidentical testosterone pellet is the best option for both men and women. The testosterone pellet is made from a plant, and it looks like the testosterone our ovaries produced when we were younger. In other words, the formula for the testosterone in the pellets looks identical to the hormones we naturally produced when we were younger, which is not the case with synthetic testosterone, such as testosterone gels and injections. The pellet works well because the level remains steady, without the lows and highs associated with other forms, including the bioidentical cream form. The steady level improves the alleviation of symptoms for a longer period of time and decreases side effects associated with testosterone.

This hormone should be handled by a physician with specialized training in hormones to ensure that the negative side effects don't occur. Negative side effects include increased facial hair, acne, thinning of hair, increased size of the clitoris, deepening of the voice, and changes in blood work. When managed and monitored appropriately, these side effects can be avoided.

I also have to remind my patients that adequate testosterone improves muscle mass and decreases the loss of muscle. Since I have started testosterone replacement, I notice that my weight is higher, however my body composition also changed. I have less fat and more muscle, which is great for metabolism and overall weight loss. I was initially frustrated after I started my testosterone pellets because I no longer saw a huge drop in pounds like I did before when eating the appropriate number of calories and making the right choices. Hence, the reason to not only monitor your weight in pounds but also monitor body composition and measure inches.

> **HOMEWORK:** Each day for two to three weeks, determine whether you are experiencing any symptoms associated with low testosterone if you are over the age of 30. If so, see a hormone specialist, to check your hormone levels and recommend a treatment plan.

SECRET #17

Estrogen

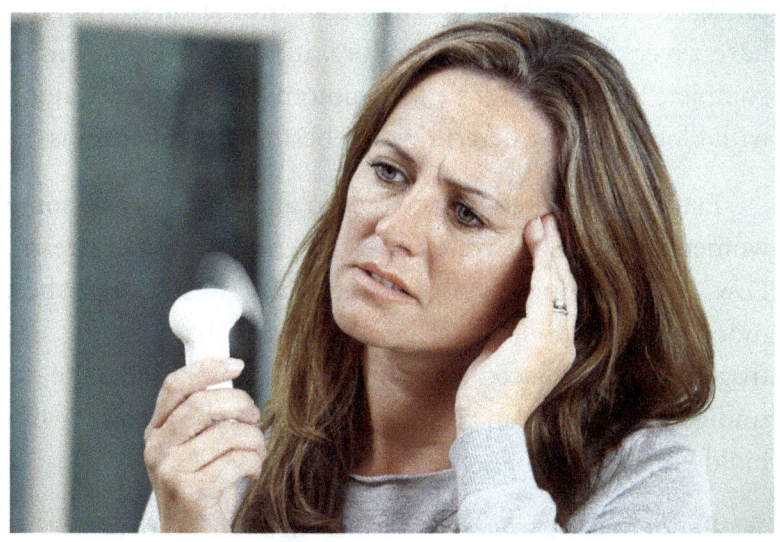

Estrogen is known as the female hormone. Estrogen levels start to decline as your ovaries start to fail and you transition into menopause. Estrogen levels vary in premenopausal women, depending on where you are in your cycle, so estrogen levels are not useful in premenopausal women who still have regular cycles or a follicle stimulating hormone (FSH) level in the premenopausal range.

If you no longer have cycles because you are in menopause, you have minimal levels of estrogen, and the best way to note whether a woman is premenopausal, postmenopausal, or perimenopausal is via a blood test called follicle stimulating hormone. FSH varies as a woman is transitioning into menopause, and may be elevated at one blood draw and lower at the next. During the transition to menopause, the estrogen levels can vary greatly, hence the reason women can have severe hot flashes. Therefore, it is necessary to give a complete history of signs and symptoms of menopause along with blood work to determine the best treatment options.

Estrogen is stored in fat, so even after menopause, some women continue to have some estrogen in the blood stream. Low and declining estrogen levels can cause hot flashes, mood changes, difficulty sleeping, fatigue, and mind fog. Estrogen can be replaced with synthetic hormones like the estradiol pill or estrogen patch, but it can also be replaced with bioidentical hormones.

Bioidentical estrogen is made from a yam plant and compressed into pellets or creams. Synthetic hormones are made from horse urine and have a different configuration compared to estrogen made by humans.

After the Women's Health Initiative study, many women stopped estrogen replacement therapy cold-turkey to treat symptoms of menopause. This randomized control study showed a slight increase in heart disease, stroke, blood clot, and cancer in women taking estradiol and/or norethindrone. However, this study included women at an average age of 60, who were starting synthetic hormones for the very first time. Synthetic hormone replacement therapy (HRT) showed a 41 percent increase in stroke, 29 percent increase in heart attacks, 26 percent increase in breast cancer and twice the rate of blood clots, as well as a 75 percent increase in Alzheimer's disease. One arm of the study took estrogen only, and another arm took estrogen and progesterone. After this study, 50 percent of family practice doctors stopped giving HRT, which significantly reduced the quality of life for millions of women. Once there was noted to be an increase in complications, the study was stopped and many women were forced to discontinue estrogen.

The study also noted a decreased risk of osteoporosis and colon cancer in the estrogen-only arm, as well as a slightly decreased risk of breast cancer in the estrogen-only group. These women had all undergone hysterectomies, so they were not required to take progesterone. Estrogen should be avoided in women with a history of a blood clot or breast cancer. Estrogen should initially be avoided in women with a history of uterine or endometrial cancer. Vaginal estrogen is a much lower dose than the other systemic options, so it may be safe to use vaginal estrogen twice a week, even with a history of cancer or blood clot, because it only works locally on vaginal tissue and does not raise blood estrogen levels. Vaginal estrogen improves vaginal atrophy and dryness, thereby improving sexual function.

So in other words, I recommend:

1. Women with a history of breast cancer, uterine cancer, and/or blood clots avoid estrogen and/or progesterone replacement therapy. However, alternative nonhormonal options are available.

2. Women under the age of 60 **without** a history of blood clot, breast cancer, or uterine cancer, and who may be experiencing moderate to severe menopausal symptoms can safely replace estrogen and progesterone (if needed) to alleviate menopausal symptoms and improve their quality of life.

3. Most women can replace testosterone safely to alleviate night sweats, fatigue, sexual dysfunction, insomnia, joint pain, mind fog, and mood changes.

> HOMEWORK: Document any symptoms you have associated with low estrogen, including hot flashes, mind fog, vaginal dryness, mood changes, difficulty sleeping, or fatigue. If significant, have your hormones checked by seeing a gynecologist who is also a hormone specialist.

SECRET #18

Thyroid

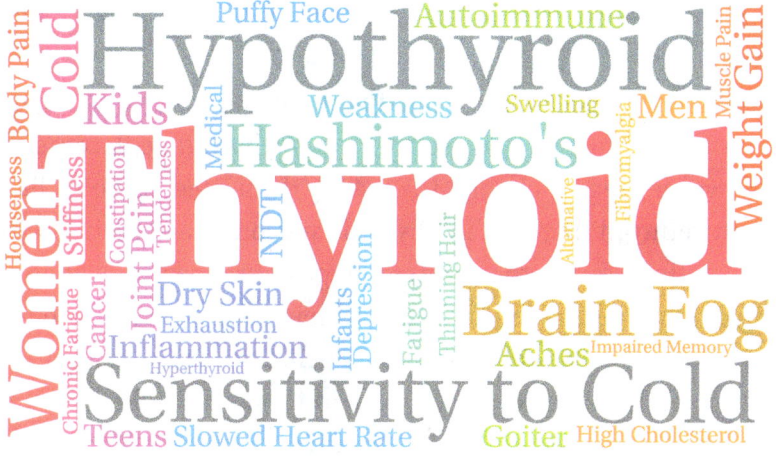

Thyroid disease can decrease your metabolism and cause you to be extremely tired and gain weight. If you are fatigued, gaining weight, depressed, cold, having memory loss, muscle aches and/or joint pain, a thyroid panel should be checked that includes a free T3, which is the most active form of thyroid hormone. Most people with low energy don't necessarily have a thyroid disorder, but it should definitely be ruled out because hypothyroidism affects up to 40 percent of women. Untreated and undertreated hypothyroidism leads to fibromyalgia, osteoporosis, Alzheimer's disease and heart disease. Most people with hypothyroidism are treated with synthetic medications like Levothyroxine and Synthroid, however, I have found that my patients have a significant improvement in symptoms when treated with dessicated thyroid like Armour thyroid and Naturethroid.

I try to ensure that my patients maintain their free T3 levels at 3.5 ng/dl to 4.2 ng/dl, which usually improves their symptoms significantly. I have had several patients with normal thyroid labs, being treated with Levothyroxine and Synthroid, which are synthetic forms of thyroid replacement. However, once I change them to a dessicated thyroid, like Naturethroid or Armour thyroid, and maintain their T3 in the optimal range, they notice a huge improvement in energy and mood, and joint pain. I have several women, who have achieved hormonal balance with pellet therapy, but they all feel better if I maintain their thyroid levels in the optimal range. Iodine and selenium optimize thyroid replacement. The goal is to optimize the thyroid levels, while still keeping thyroid levels in the normal range, because high levels can damage the heart and cause palpitations, jitteriness, and increased anxiety.

> **HOMEWORK:** Document any symptoms associated with thyroid disease such as fatigue, weight gain, depression, cold intolerance, memory loss, muscle aches, or joint pain. If you notice these symptoms consistently, see a physician who specializes in hormone balance and uses natural thyroid options.

SECRET #19

Weight Gain

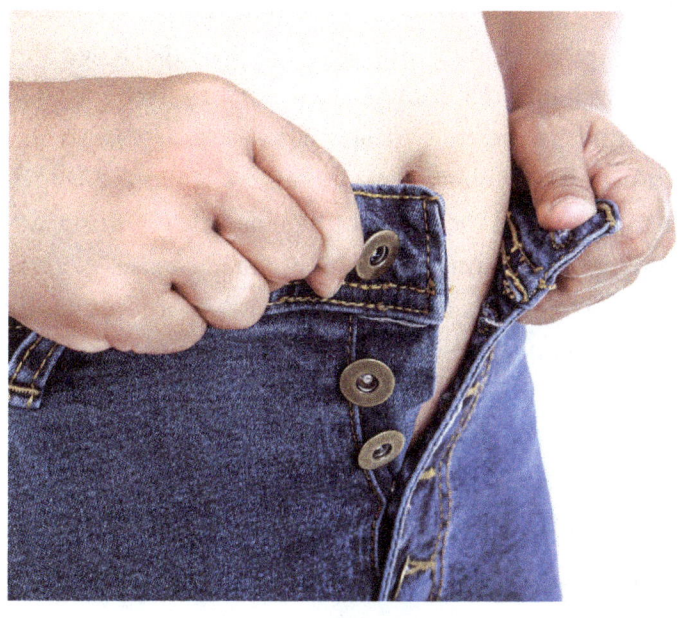

As women transition into menopause, many notice an increase in weight because hormonal imbalance definitely affects weight. Women transitioning into menopause can gain 5 to 15 pounds with no change in eating habits or exercise. Hormonal balance can help increase muscle and decrease fat, which makes weight loss and maintenance much easier. Women tend to gain weight because they are suffering from insomnia. Not sleeping increases cortisol levels, which increases weight. Also, because women are more tired and irritable during this time, many women will self-medicate with comfort food and sweet snacks to feel better. Also during this time, because of significant mood changes, many women will start taking antidepressants, which may increase appetite and weight. Some women initially start to experience this weight gain well before menopause, secondary to the decline in testosterone in the mid to late 30s. After assessing and treating hormonal imbalance most women can lose the added weight and control their weight with calorie counting, accountability, portion control, frequent small meals, exercise and adequate water. It is necessary to weigh more frequently during this challenging time, although with testosterone replacement, you may not notice a large drop in pounds when trying to lose weight. A body composition analysis would be another way to measure weight control along with measurements of the waist, thighs, hips, and arms.

The added muscle does add a few pounds, so I remind my patients to not only focus on their weight in pounds, but also to monitor inches and body composition, which will show fat and water percentage, as well as muscle mass. As long as you are losing fat and maintaining or gaining muscle, you are headed in the right direction.

HOMEWORK: Weigh yourself daily, have a body composition analysis, and follow my secrets to maintaining a healthy weight. If you notice difficulty maintaining your weight, see a gynecologist who specializes in hormone therapy and weight loss.

SECRET #20

Mood

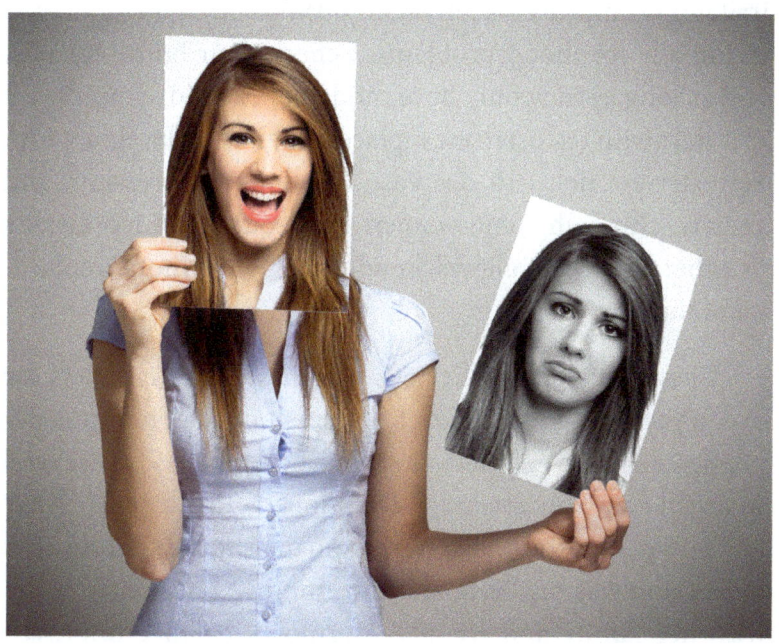

Up to 30 percent of women going through menopause experience increased depression, irritability, and anxiety. Well before menopause, women with low testosterone levels, which can start in the late 20s to early 30s, may experience anxiety, irritability and/or depression. Hormonal balance can help to improve mood significantly. Many of my patients with known depression and anxiety notice that it worsens during the menopausal transition. However, after hormonal balance, many of my patients' symptoms improve back to baseline, or they completely resolve. Some of my patients become more irritable because of lack of sleep, so they are just more tired and irritable. By improving sleep through hormone balance, irritability improves significantly. When my patients come in initially for mood problems, I check their hormone labs, and as long as they only have moderate or mild symptoms, I will start with testosterone replacement if their levels are low. Testosterone helps to decrease irritability, depression, and anxiety, although some women still require antidepressants or other mood stabilizers in addition to hormone replacement therapy.

I have a patient in her 60s who has been on pellets for over a year. Prior to the pellet, she spent most of her time depressed and in bed. She was seeing a psychiatrist for several years and was on several medications with no relief. After her first pellet, she was a new woman! She had energy, her depression was resolved, and this improved her relationship with her family and friends! Hormonal balance improved her mood symptoms so much that her psychiatrist called me to see how I treated her because she saw her miraculous recovery. She continues to take some of her psyche medications, and along with balanced hormones, she has regained her life. So although hormonal balance may not get everyone completely off their antidepressants and other mood stabilizers, it improves quality of life and mood significantly!

> **HOMEWORK:** Document any symptoms associated with your mood, sleep, appetite, energy, and concentration. If you notice that you are consistently having symptoms that affect your quality of life, or you have a family history of mental illness, see a healthcare provider. Preferably a gynecologist who specializes in hormonal balance to increase your treatment options. Also, seek out a therapist that you can see at least once a month.

SECRET #21

Sex Drive

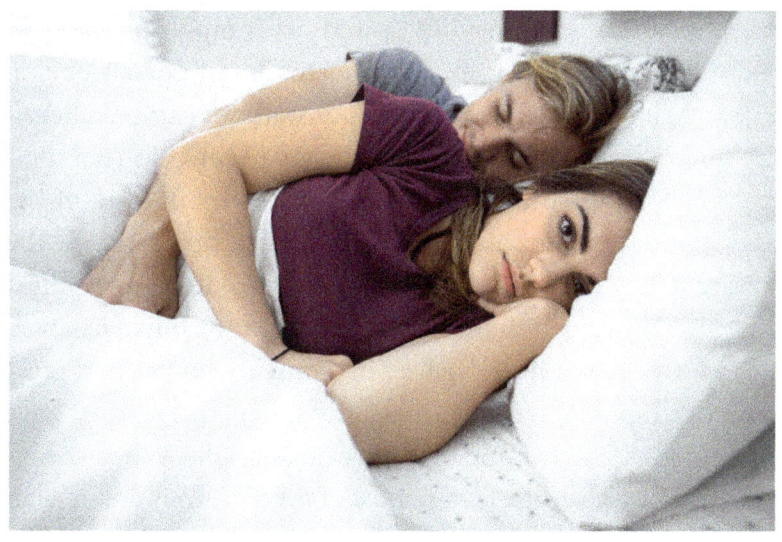

Many women with hormonal imbalances experience a significant decrease in sex drive and orgasms. Some women with low estrogen experience vaginal dryness and pain with intercourse, which can decrease sex drive and orgasms. Women may experience a decrease in sex drive secondary to low testosterone levels caused by birth control or the natural decline in testosterone with age. Low sex drive can cause problems in marriages and relationships, while healthy sex improves health and quality of life.

Many of my patients over the age of 35, and sometimes much younger, experience a decline in libido and orgasms. Libido for women is dependent not only on balanced hormones but overall energy and health and the stability of the relationship. Many times, women are just overwhelmed with their personal responsibilities and are simply too tired to think about sex. Low sex drive related to fatigue and being overwhelmed with too many responsibilities can be relieved by finding ways to get more rest and decreasing some of their responsibilities so they are not exhausted by the end of the day. Sometimes marital/relationship bliss can decrease the desire to have sex, which can be improved with couple's therapy and better communication in the relationship. However, I have worked with a large set of women who are in a great relationship and are not necessarily fatigued. Yet, they have little to no sex drive; and they have no idea why. When checking their testosterone levels, most of the time they are in what we consider the normal lab range. However, I find that by increasing their total testosterone levels to 80 to 150 ng/dl, they have a significant increase in sex drive and orgasm. Sex drive starts to decline well before natural menopause sets in. Testosterone is the first hormone to decline as we age, therefore many women complain about sex drive years before they transition into menopause. Often antidepressants and other medications can decrease sex drive and orgasm. Sometimes, changing these medications can help improve libido tremendously.

> **HOMEWORK:** Pay attention to your libido and sexual function. Have a conversation with your partner and determine if your libido or sexual function has changed. If so, have your hormones balanced and see a sex therapist if necessary.

SECTION 4

Visiting Your Gynecologist/ Prevention

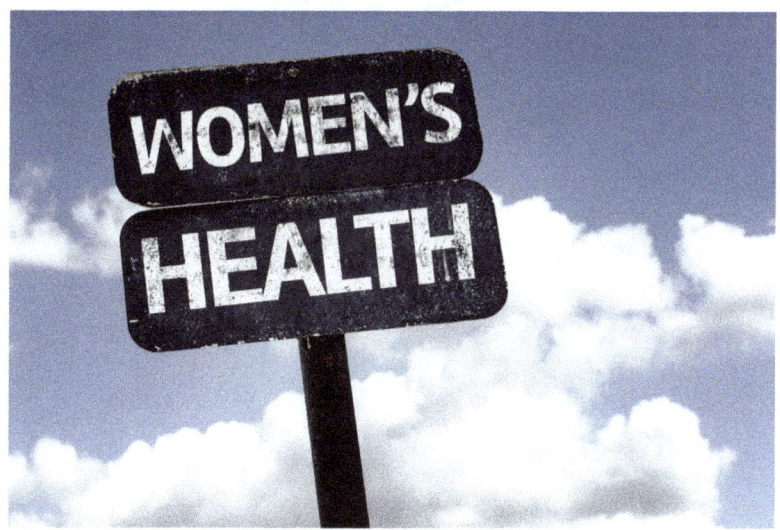

One of our duties to maintaining our total wellness and living our best lives is to have our preventive exams. You should have a gynecological exam annually if you are under the age of 65 and you should also see your primary care doctor annually for a preventive exam. It is necessary to have your normal screenings and understand your risks and numbers so that you can maintain your health. Having your annual exams will allow you to take any preventive measures that may improve your health so you can live well and age beautifully.

SECRET #22

Pap Smear Recommendations and Annual Exams

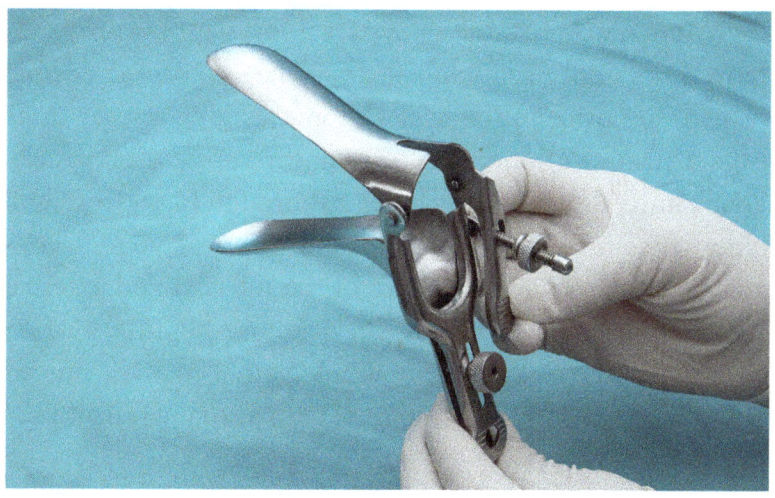

A pap smear is a small part of a woman's annual exam. This occurs when the speculum is placed and a sample is taken from the cervix then sent to a pathology lab to ensure that the cells are normal. Women are exposed to human papilloma virus (HPV) at some point in life, and HPV can cause cervical cancer. The pap smear prevents cervical cancer because it shows abnormal cells that we watch more closely to ensure they regress back to normal, instead of progressing to cancer, which takes several years. Pap smears are performed on women, starting at the age of 21, every one to five years, depending on risk factors and history. Pap smears prevent cervical cancer if done regularly and are only a small part of your annual exam. You should have an annual exam yearly and your gynecologist will decide if a pap smear is necessary based on your history.

Women who have had a hysterectomy with the cervix removed may not need pap smears if they had three normal pap smears prior to the hysterectomy, as long as they don't have a history of abnormal pap smears or cervical cancer. Your annual exam also includes a thorough history, weight, blood pressure, breast exam, examination of your ovaries and uterus, as well as an exam of the internal and external vagina. During this exam, I can diagnose fibroids, ovarian cysts, vulvar cysts, and other pathology that could be missed without regular exams. I also screen for sexually transmitted infections if necessary.

When visiting the gynecologist, it is important to have all of your concerns written before your appointment so that all of your questions are answered. An annual gynecology exam is a great time to ensure that you are living a healthy lifestyle. I encourage my patients to maintain a healthy weight and to adopt behaviors that will decrease their risk of heart disease and cancer. I recommend that you start mammograms at the age of 40 and have them yearly. Some choose to go every two years, although I only recommend this if you don't have obvious risk factors for breast cancer. If you have a first-degree relative diagnosed with breast cancer, I recommend you have a baseline mammogram at the age of 35 and yearly mammograms starting at age of 40. I recommend you have a colonoscopy, which prevents colon cancer starting at age of 50, unless you have a family history of colon cancer and then I recommend you have your first colonoscopy five years before your first-degree relative was diagnosed with colon cancer. Bone density screenings should be performed in women aged 65 and older or earlier with risk factors such as previous fracture, long-term steroid therapy, parental history of hip fracture, low body weight, cigarette smoking, excessive alcohol consumption, and arthritis, to name a few. I recommend you have a thorough heart work-up at the age of 50, and sometimes earlier, if you have a strong family history of heart disease, are experiencing symptoms like shortness of breath, chest pain, or leg swelling, or if you went through menopause before the age of 50. Your heart starts to age when the ovaries are removed, or when your ovaries naturally stop producing hormones, which can be easily shown with a blood test, along with menopausal symptoms. I still recommend you have a primary care physician to manage your non-gynecologic health issues.

> **HOMEWORK:** Make sure you have had all recommended screenings for your age and history; if not, schedule all necessary appointments to ensure that you are preventing disease to the best of your ability.

SECRET #23

Fibroids/Bleeding

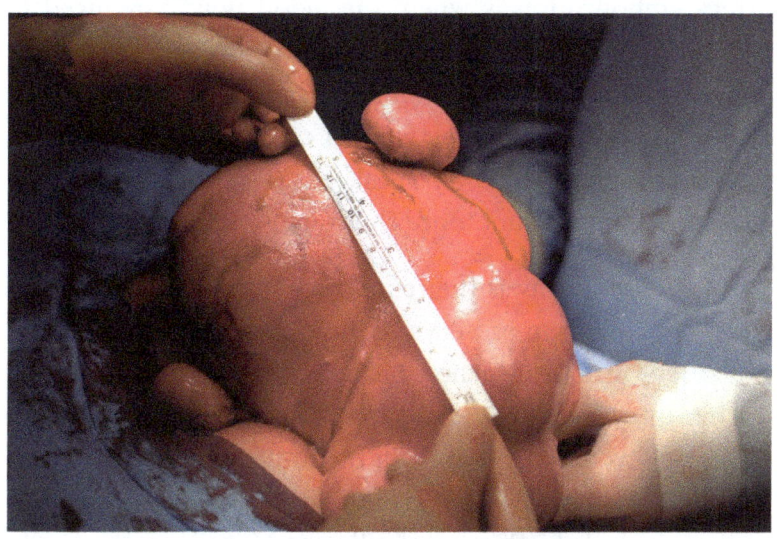

Fibroids are benign tumors of the uterus, and are one of the most common abnormalities in gynecology, affecting 80 to 90 percent of all women over the age of 30. Fibroids can be completely asymptomatic or they can cause pain, abnormal bleeding, fertility problems, pain with intercourse, difficulty with urination, or constipation. They may become large enough to cause pelvic pressure.

Fibroids do not cause cancer and don't always require surgery. When fibroids are small and asymptomatic, they can be managed more conservatively. Treatment options for symptomatic fibroids include hormones, uterine artery embolization, hysteroscopy with myosure, abdominal myomectomy, endometrial ablation (burning the lining of the uterus to stop bleeding), and of course, hysterectomy. A uterine artery embolization is where the blood flow is reduced to decrease the amount of bleeding from fibroids. It does not help significantly with size or pain, but definitely decreases blood loss. Although some women can still get pregnant after a uterine artery embolization, it is not recommended for women who may want more children.

A myomectomy is the removal of fibroids while leaving the uterus intact to preserve fertility. This can be done as an outpatient procedure where a camera is placed through the vagina into the uterus. Next, an instrument is used to remove polyps and fibroids from the lining to decrease bleeding, and possibly improve fertility. Several other noninvasive options include birth control pills, the NuvaRing, the Ortho Evra patch, Depo-Provera, Lupron, Mirena, and the NEXPLANON. These hormones are used to control symptoms associated with fibroids in women not actively trying to get pregnant. Another option is a medication called Triaminic acid, which is nonhormonal and decreases bleeding associated with heavy cycles. I see several women who come in for a second opinion because they have been told they need a hysterectomy or major surgery due to their fibroids. Whereas sometimes I agree with those recommendations, there are several women who I have treated conservatively. These women were able to avoid a major surgery and were still relieved of their symptoms while also preserving their uterus.

> **HOMEWORK:** Make sure you have your annual exam this year. If you have fibroids, monitor your symptoms, which include heavy bleeding, pain during cycles or pelvic pain outside of cycles, pain with intercourse, irregular bleeding, and/or changes in urination or bowel movement patterns. Be sure to discuss your findings with your doctor.

SECRET #24

Finished Having Babies, Now What?

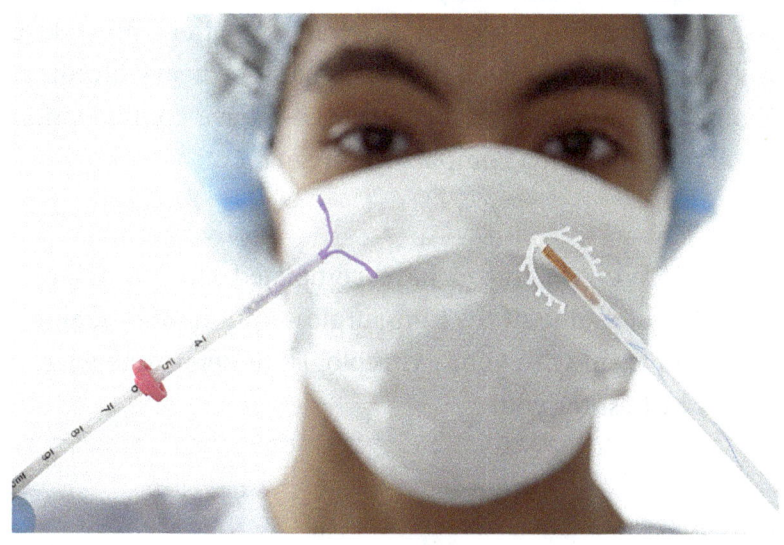

Once you have completed childbearing, it's not necessary to have a tubal ligation, which requires an outpatient surgery. Now, there are several long-term, noninvasive options that are just as effective with fewer risks, including the intrauterine devices (IUDs), the NEXPLANON, and a male vasectomy, which is an office procedure that your spouse can undergo to prevent your pregnancy. There is also an office-based procedure that can be done without general anesthesia, called an essure tubal. All of these options are 99.9 percent effective. Many women over the age of 35 who don't smoke can continue the birth control pill, ring, or patch. Hormonal birth control for five years actually decreases the risk of ovarian and endometrial cancer. Some women choose to have a tubal ligation because they want to avoid hormones. Others may have heavy cycles and need an outpatient procedure called an ablation, which decreases or stops heavy bleeding. Women undergoing an ablation MUST have contraception in place to prevent a complicated pregnancy.

> **HOMEWORK:** If you have completed child bearing, investigate some of the non-surgical options above, and discuss them with your gynecologist to determine what may be best for you!

SECRET #25

Adolescents and the Gynecologist

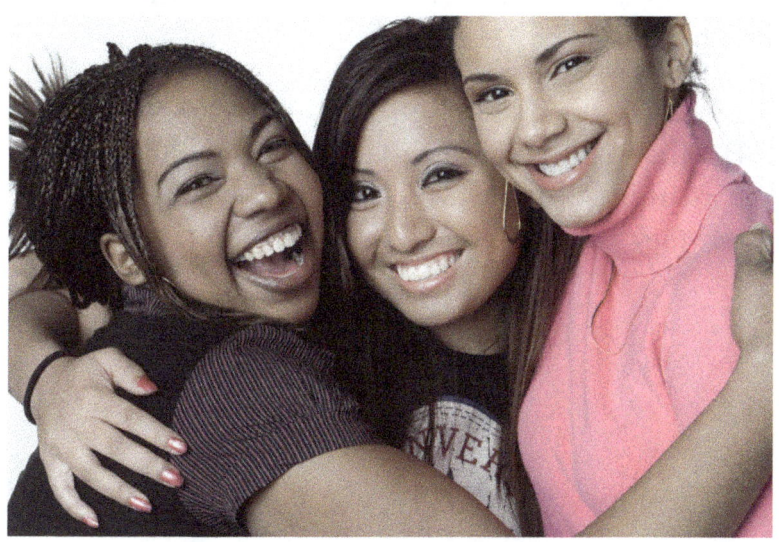

The American College of Obstetricians and Gynecologists recommend that adolescents start seeing a gynecologist between the ages of 13 and 15 years old. If your adolescent has problems with her cycle or other female issues before then, it is reasonable to see a gynecologist earlier. Before the age of 21, most adolescents don't need an uncomfortable vaginal exam because most adolescent screenings can be done through urine. When I see adolescents, I educate them about their bodies, proper hygiene, normal body changes, abstinence, condoms, and wellness, including healthy living and weight management. This is a great age to start teaching our adolescents to grow up and become healthy adults. Wellness is learned; it is not innate. The earlier we encourage healthy behaviors in our children, the more likely they are to become healthy adults.

> HOMEWORK: Share with some of your friends the importance of their adolescents seeing a gynecologist before they are 15 years old.

SECRET #26

Vaginal Maintenance

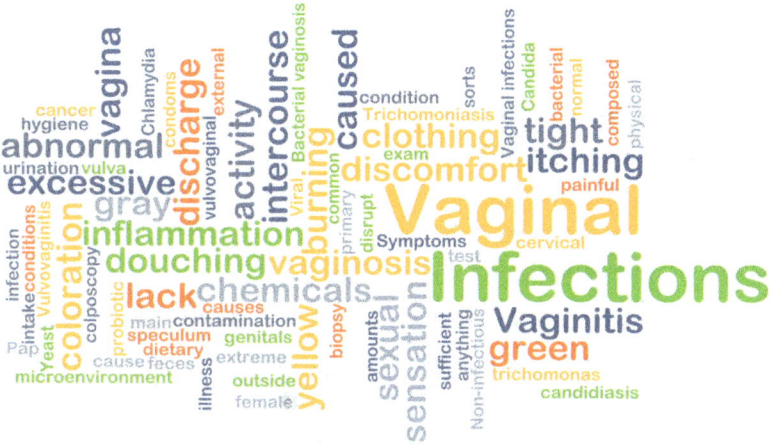

I find that a lot of adolescent girls and women are very concerned with vaginal odor and hygiene. I recommend that my Belles use plain ole water and, if necessary, a very mild soap to clean. I recommend to avoid anything with perfumes or fragrances like the namebrand vaginal hygiene products, including cleansers, pH balance, and many of the lubricants. I usually recommend organic coconut oil As a lubricant, I recommend Dove white bar sensitive skin soap or Dove unscented bar soap for vaginal cleansing, because they do not alter vaginal pH balance. Many of the other cleansing products have perfumes, dyes, and other irritants. These products can alter pH balance, leading to undesirable yeast infections and/or bacterial vaginosis. As you know, yeast can cause a thick, cottage cheese discharge, odor, and severe itching and irritation. Bacterial vaginosis is caused by an increase in vaginal pH, which can be caused by perfumes, dyes, and irritants, as well as sperm. Clean with water and a mild white bar soap, not shower gels and liquids because they tend to have perfumes, dyes, and other irritants that change the normal flora of the vagina. Bacterial vaginosis can cause a grey-like discharge with a very fishy odor, which can be more noticeable after menstrual bleeding and intercourse. Bacterial vaginosis and yeast are not sexually transmitted infections, but sexually transmitted infections can also cause a change in vaginal discharge and color, pelvic pain, fever, and painful intercourse. So do not assume you have bacterial vaginosis or a yeast infection until you have been given a diagnosis from your physician. Also, make sure to have sexually transmitted infections ruled out by your physician if you are sexually active."

HOMEWORK: Make sure you are using a mild white soap and avoiding irritants like shower gels, perfumes, and bubble baths. Purchase hypoallergenic baby wipes to be used for cleansing the vaginal area between showers to prevent vaginal odor.

SECRET #27

Breast Cancer

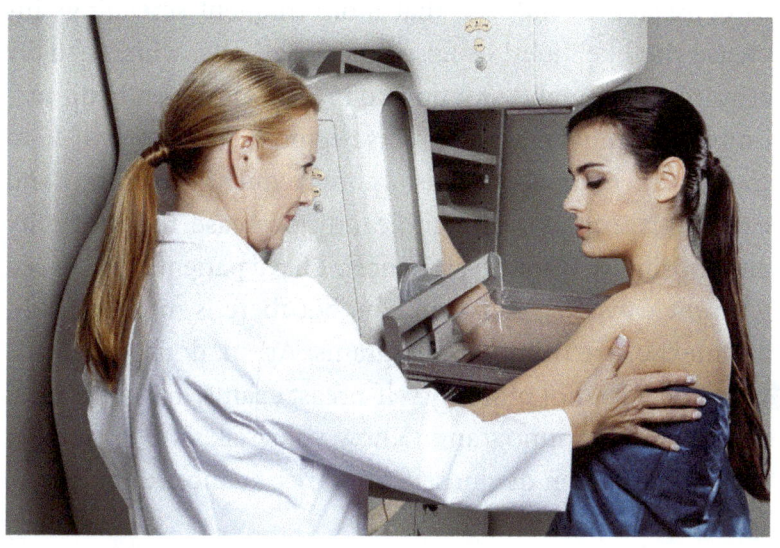

Breast cancer is the number one cancer cause of death for women. Women should start having mammograms at the age of 40 or earlier if there is a significant family history of breast cancer or risk factors associated with breast cancer. Risk factors for breast cancer include increasing age, obesity after menopause, increased alcohol consumption of two to five drinks per day, early puberty and late menopause, family history of breast cancer, and long-term use of birth control pills. There have been new recommendations regarding the frequency and the age to start breast cancer screenings. I still recommend monthly breast exams and annual clinical exams. Breast cancer screening has become a controversial topic,—some experts recommend starting at 45 to 50 years of age and only having them every other year. This appears to be related to the idea that more frequent screenings increase the likelihood of false positive results, which usually require a thorough work up and biopsy. However, I still recommend annual mammograms beginning at the age of 40 to most of my patients because more frequent screenings and earlier screenings can significantly decrease the mortality and morbidity from breast cancer. I have patients concerned with their exposure to radiation, but there is minimal radiation exposure from mammograms. Again, don't underestimate the power of monthly self-breast exams, annual clinical exams, and mammograms. Know your risk, and remember that most women diagnosed with breast cancer don't have a family history.

> **HOMEWORK:** Do monthly self-breast exams, have an annual exam with your gynecologist, and have an annual mammogram starting at the age of 40.

SECRET #28

Heart Disease

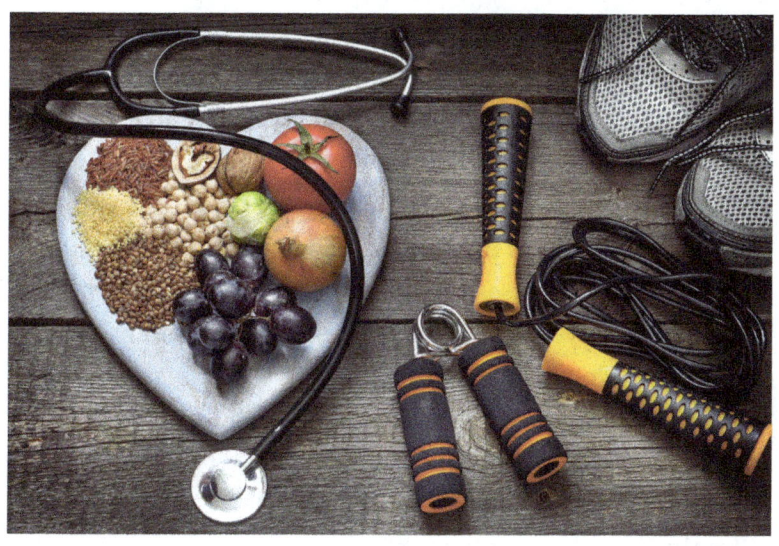

Did you know that heart disease is the number one killer of men and women in the United States? To prevent heart disease, it is necessary to first maintain a healthy weight, which is a body mass index less than 25, choose healthy diet options, such as lean protein, fiber, and five servings of fruits and vegetables daily. Also, minimize saturated fat, avoid trans fat, and eat healthy fat like unsaturated fats found in avocado, almonds, pistachios, and other nuts, as well as olives and olive oil.

A family history of heart disease before the age of 50 to 55 in a first-degree relative increases your risk for heart disease. A personal history of high blood pressure, high cholesterol, and diabetes all increase your risk of heart disease as well, and don't forget the silent killer: uncontrolled high blood pressure. It is imperative that you see your primary care doctor regularly for screening and prevention. If you are taking medications to control your blood pressure, it is very important to monitor your blood pressure regularly and take your blood pressure medications as prescribed. The goal is to maintain your blood pressure to be less than 125/80 mmHg. Exercise also decreases your risk of heart disease, improves weight and metabolism, and helps with overall energy and well-being. Not only is it important to include cardiovascular exercise like walking, running, biking, swimming, and interval training, you should also remember your resistance training exercises. Supplements like omega -3, CoQ10 and Vitamin D3 help improve cardiac health.

I recommend all my ladies have a cardiac work-up by the time they reach menopause, and earlier if necessary when there is a personal and/or family history of heart disease, stroke, or high blood pressure. Of equal importance, if my patients have a history of chronic fatigue, snoring, or insomnia, I encourage them to have a sleep study to rule out sleep apnea. Remember, sleep apnea can play a large role in heart disease if not treated. This is because the stress on your heart from uncontrolled sleep apnea can significantly increase your risk of heart disease and death.

> **HOMEWORK:** See a primary care doctor, have a baseline cardiovascular work-up if you are menopausal (surgical or natural), investigate your family history to better understand your risk factors for heart disease and improve your risk by maintaining a healthy blood pressure.

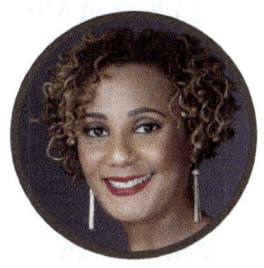

About the Author

Dr. Mia Cowan is a board-certified gynecologist with special training in physician-directed weight loss and hormonal balance for men and women. Her mission is to help women, known as her "Ageless Belles," who are struggling with weight gain, fatigue, and low sex drive, improve their B3: beauty, balance, and belief, through education and cutting-edge medicine (programs, media, speaking, blogs, and books) so they can live well and age beautifully.

Dr. Mia earned her Bachelor of Science in biology and a Master of Arts in health education and promotion from the University of Alabama. She went on to complete her Doctor of Medicine and residency training in obstetrics and gynecology from the Medical College of Wisconsin and a Master of Business Administration at Auburn University. Over the last several years, she has been the recipient of several awards, including the 2013 Best in Minority Business Award for Outstanding Young Professionals and the 2013 Shades Valley YMCA Adult Volunteer Award, and she was named one of Birmingham Business Journals' Top 40 Under 40 and Who's Who in Black Alabama Top 20 under 40.

Dr. Mia currently resides in Birmingham, Alabama, with her husband, Joseph, and their two children, Marley and Jamil. In her spare time, she enjoys serving on the health ministry at church, traveling, reading, snorkeling, spending time with family and friends, and writing.

To connect, visit her website at **miacowanmd.com**

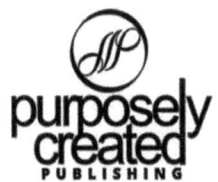

CREATING DISTINCTIVE BOOKS
WITH INTENTIONAL RESULTS

We're a collaborative group of creative masterminds with a mission to produce high-quality books to position you for monumental success in the marketplace.

Our professional team of writers, editors, designers, and marketing strategists work closely together to ensure that every detail of your book is a clear representation of the message in your writing.

Want to know more?
Write to us at info@publishyourgift.com
or call (888) 949-6228

Discover great books, exclusive offers, and more at
www.PublishYourGift.com

Connect with us on social media

@publishyourgift

www.ingramcontent.com/pod-product-compliance
Lightning Source LLC
Chambersburg PA
CBHW070030040426
42333CB00040B/1424